MW01166694

Managing Gout and Coping With Gout

A reference for gout sufferers including gout diet.

by

George Groddington and Robert Rymore

1

Table of Contents

Table of Contents

Table of Contents

Table of Contents

Chapter 1: Introduction

1) Brief History

Gout; the disease of distinction. A frequently mismanaged and neglected disease, gout has enjoyed special attention over the centuries. Egyptians were the first to identify Gout in 2640 BC. Evidence of gout was found in 4000 year old Egyptian mummies.

The first written description of gout was attributed to Hippocrates, who wrote it as "podagra". It is understood that this term existed well before him. He regarded gout as being the result of an excessive accumulation of one of the four bodily humors. The 4 humors are bloodstream, phlegm, the yellow bile and the African American bile. It was thought that probably the excess of phlegm is responsible for triggering gout.

The human body has a unique system of stability. This system manifests itself in different forms in different positions, conditions and scenarios. For example, if you are standing upright, this system can be identified as a balance required to do so. A static equilibrium of the human body provides this balance and we can stand upright. Similarly, in homeostasis, the body maintains a stable internal environment. A group of positive and negative feedback mechanisms help the body in maintaining that internal stability vital to health.

Some of the most prevalent diseases resulting from failure of the body to maintain homeostasis are:
-Diabetes,
-Dehydration,
-Hypoglycemia,
-Hyperglycemia &
-Gout

In addition to the above, any disease caused by the presence of a toxin in the bloodstream can also be attributed to disturbances in homeostasis.

This book exclusively addresses gout and provides a medical and social perspective to treat it effectively. In doing so, it touches upon cultural, moral and personal effects the disease produces. Practical information that can help patients suffering from gout is the hall mark of this book.

2) Why Do We Get Gout?

The uric acid pool size of an adult male is about 1,200 mg. About 700 mg is produced daily and it is mainly excreted by the kidneys (70-72%/500 mg) and some excretion is through feces (28-30%/200 mg). So excretion keeps the urate levels within the pool size. According to the mechanisms, hyperuricemia is classified into over-production and under-excretion.

Over-production of urate is caused by:
-PRPP synthetase super-activity (a regulatory enzyme in purine and pyrimidine biosynthesis; enhanced activity of this enzyme results in an increase in purine biosynthesis leading to gout).
-HPRT deficiency (Deficiency of hypoxanthine-guanine phosphoribosyltransferase (HPRT). This is an error, an inborn error of purine metabolism that is associated with gout.
-Leukemia
-Alcohol ingestion.
Under-excretion of urate is caused by:
-Renal insufficiency and
-Diuretic treatment.

The hyperuricemia cascade is triggered by various factors including dietary intake of purines, tissue nucleic acid and endogenous purine synthesis, which leads to excess formation of urate or uric acid, the end product of purine metabolism.
This excessive urate formation triggers over-production and under-excretion leading to hyperuricemia. This condition further

facilitates silent tissue deposition, renal manifestation, cardiovascular events, gout and mortality.

As treatment of gout primarily depends upon medications and certain changes in lifestyle, this book makes a conscious effort to explain these two factors in detail. At the same time, it uncovers ravaging side effects of the majority of medications used for managing pain in gout and in doing so explains the recent shift toward alternative remedies.

Chapter 2: Prevalence & Risk Factors for Gout

1) Prevalence of Gout

Gout and its precursor Hyperuricemia is one of the most commonly occurring diseases in the west nowadays and many studies have demonstrated that the incidence of Gout has increased because of mismanagement. Irrespective of the fact that it is completely curable.

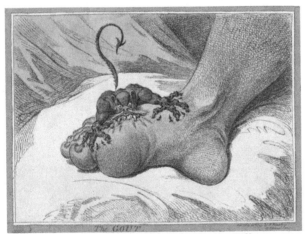

Source: "The gout james gillray" by James Gillray - http://commons.wikimedia.org

Findings gathered from the United States National Health and Nutrition Examination Survey (NHANES III) have indicated that gout incidence is on the rise.
The data collected from NHANES 2007-2008 shows the occurrence of gout in the US has increased in the most recent twenty years and now influences over 8.3 million (4%) of the American population. The stats reveal a prevalence rate of 5.9% in males and 2.0% among females.

10

The possibilities of Hyperuricemia have also increased, influencing 43.3 million (21%) grown-ups in the U.S. These findings conclude that over the past two decades Gout has increased by 1.2% and Hyperuricemia by 3.2%. The increase is associated with obesity, metabolic disorder, and hypertension. Increase in prevalence in several other countries like China, New Zeeland and Africa have similar associations.

2) Risk Factors

Medical studies and research have now given a new dimension to the role of uric acid in the human body and its estimation in patients with Gout. Uric acid was formerly known as a nitrogenous waste product of metabolism eliminated from kidneys and bowels. The biological functions of uric acid observed after several scientific studies challenged this non-functional theory. Data collected from various clinical findings and researches link salt retention, hypertension, hyper-triglyceridemia, cardiovascular events and obesity to high uric acid levels in body.

Studies show that changes in diet, life style and medications have great impact on longevity and reduction of severity of symptoms in Gout. However modifiable and non-modifiable risk factors exist for Hyperuricemia and Gout. Modifiable risk factors can be changed by taking correct measures against them while non-modifiable factors can't be changed. People who suffer from high serum concentration of uric acid often develop metabolic disorders which further make a chain of health problems like low "good" cholesterol, high blood pressure, kidney problems and a reduced quality of life. It is well understood now which factors increase the chances of gout and which steps can reduce its prevalence. A better understanding of these factors will allow sufferers and caregivers to reduce gout's impact.

a) Non-Modifiable Risk Factors

Age
Middle-Aged Adults: Middle aged men in their mid-40's have a great tendency of developing Gout. High alcohol consumption, obesity, high blood pressure, and low "good" cholesterol levels are characteristic features of this group.

Elderly: Old men and women have equal tendencies for developing gout. Due to deposition of urate crystals in the kidney leading to renal impairment and use of diuretics, this group is prone to develop Gout.

Children: It is not common in children. They are only likely to develop Gout if there are certain genetic disorders. In such cases, the condition is referred to as Juvenile Gout.

Gender
Men/Males: The incidence of developing Gout is more common in men as compared to women. The uric acid level starts rising in puberty and exceeds 7mg/dl in 5-8% of men indicating Hyperuricemia. Hyperuricemia when not properly treated in time, may lead to development of Gout in 20-40 years. So technically, men who develop gout in later stages of life experience first attacks in their twenties and early thirties.

Women/Females: Estrogen plays a vital role of antagonizing uric acid from the body by facilitating its excretion by the kidney. Menopausal women are at high risk of developing Gout. Several reports suggest that there are only 15% chances for women to develop Gout before menopause. By the age of 60 men and women have equal tendencies to develop Gout. Studies suggest that at age 80 women develop Gout more often than men.

Genetics
People with a family history of gout have a 20% chance of suffering from the disease. Uric acid concentration in blood serum

levels is inheritable. Genetic studies show that genes that encode proteins to eliminate urate via the kidney can be a risk factor to develop gout. Mutations in these genes increase risk of gout three to five folds because these alterations reduce elimination of uric acid from the body causing Hyperuricemia. Lesch–Nyhan syndrome (LNS), also known as juvenile gout, is a rare inherited disorder which occurs as a result of a decrease in the enzyme hypoxanthine-guanine phosphoribosyl-transferase (HGPRT). This deficiency increases the overall concentration of uric acid in the body, resulting in Hyperuricemia.

b) Modifiable Risk Factors

Obesity/Overweight
Obesity doubles the likelihood of gout, as poor eating habits causing obesity serve a pathway to developing gout. The higher the body mass index (BMI), the higher the likelihood of gout occurring will be. Fructose consumption aids in gout development and even if someone does not develop gout, increased uric acid levels irritate the blood vessel lining, which is the first step towards strokes and cardiovascular events. Production of Nitrous oxide, a gas which allows blood vessels to relax, is also inhibited by uric acid thus causing high blood pressure. In this way a high uric acid level in the body causes hypertension.

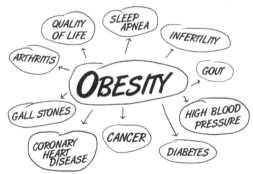

The prevalence of obese children developing gout at puberty is much higher. Risk could be reduced by taking a low calorie diet and exercise. Traditionally, gout was considered the disease of the rich but its increase incidence in low middle classes shows the association with obesity and diabetes.

Joint injuries
Injury of the joints as a result of an accident could predispose to gout if not treated adequately. Surgeries also contribute to gout, as the body fluid level of uric acid is disturbed causing Hyperuricemia. The uric acid is accumulated in injured joints and triggers gout. Trauma initiates a small event of inflammatory process, which further initiates gouty arthritis in that particular joint. It may take a year or two for the symptoms of gout to appear in the affected/injured joint. Quick treatment of injuries can certainly prevent development of gout.

Infections
Infection can also trigger a series of inflammatory processes leading to gout. Swelling and redness in joints caused by infection is referred to as septic arthritis, infectious arthritis or bacterial arthritis. If one large joint like the hip or knee is affected, it can spread to multiple joints in a very short time. An open wound or opening due to surgical procedure could trigger infection. The foreign invaders when entered in the body infect joints and cause inflammation. Bacteria such as Haemophilus influenza, staphylococcus and streptococcus cause septic arthritis in adults and children. Virus induced infections include hepatitis A,B & C, herpes virus, HIV(AIDS)virus and mumps, while fungi may also contributes to the development of inflammation.

Occupation
Work and leisure activities have a great influence on muscle and joint injuries and can predispose people in their life to gout and arthritis. Heavy lifting, kneeling and squatting for a prolonged period of time can damage and deteriorate cartilage. Sport such as football, baseball and soccer also induce gouty arthritis.

Following a simple and moderate exercise routine is good for everyone and helps in reducing the risk of gout. While walking and jogging neither trigger gout, they also don't prevent it.

3) Managing Hyperuricemia

Studies suggest that 60% of patients suffering from acute gout feel episodes of severe pain in a period of six months. It is therefore suggested that those patients who only have a mild attack of gout once in a year should change their lifestyle and eating habits to prevent it instead of going for a long-term therapy. But, if it does not reduce or control symptoms and pain, then one must start treatment. As a part of therapeutic measures in gout, patients must be educated and should be well informed of diet, proper management, and lifestyle changes necessary to subside pain and improve the quality of life.

a) Dietary Measures & Improving Quality Of Life

Avoid following:
- Red or organ meat, which is rich in purine content
- Corn syrups, sweetened sodas other beverages or foods rich in fructose
- High consumption of alcohol

Limit following:
- Limit the serving size of beef, lamb and other red meat and sea food, especially shell fish and sardines
- Beer and alcohol
- Naturally sweet fruit juices, table sugar, sweetened beverages and desserts
- Table salts, sauces and gravies

Encourage following:
- Dairy products with low fat
- Vegetables
- Regular exercise

- Smoking cessation (say no to smoking as it can lead to multiple health hazards and increase complications)
- Drinking plenty of water.

b) Decision to treat Hyperuricemia

The purpose of medicines is preventing acute attacks by reducing pain and inflammation. Treatment also aims at preventing future attacks by lowering the overall uric acid burden in body. Drug therapy becomes essential when there are acute gout attacks and tophus is diagnosed.

Asymptomatic Hyperuricemia
The condition where there are elevated levels of uric acid in the blood but the patient develops no signs of crystal deposition or gout is referred to as asymptomatic gout or asymptomatic Hyperuricemia. Its treatment has some risk along with it, and it is not successful in many cases.

Symptomatic Hyperuricemia
Diagnosis of gout, uric acid stones or uric acid nephropathy calls for initiation of therapy.

Acute Gouty Arthritis
The following medicines are used alone or in combination to prevent acute gout attacks:
- Non-steroidal Anti-inflammatory drugs (NSAIDs),
- Colchicines
- Corticosteroids.

Non-steroidal Anti-inflammatory Drugs (NSAIDs)
NSAIDs are for acute gout attacks especially in youngsters with no serious health issues. Many over-the-counter NSAIDs provide fast relief including ibuprofen, naproxen, and ketoprofen. While others like Indomethacin is a prescription NSAID. Indomethacin and other NSAIDs are prescribed approximately for 7-10 days or for a longer duration until the pain subsides. NSAIDs can cause

gastrointestinal discomfort and ulcers and instructions should be strictly followed for how much and how long one can take in order to avoid serious side effects. NSAIDs should be used with caution in patients with peptic ulcer disease and renal insufficiencies. Diabetic patients who take oral anti-diabetic medicines should adjust the dose to avoid possible drug interaction.

Colchicines
Derived from a plant known as alkaloid colchicines, it has the ability to exhibit highly anti-inflammatory activities. It is used to prevent gout attacks as a prophylaxis for recurrent attacks. NSAIDs have replaced colchicines currently because of its extreme side effects and intolerance. Caution should be taken in the elderly and patients with kidney, liver or bone marrow problems. It effects fertility and hence should not be given in pregnancy.

Corticosteroids
Corticosteroids, known as steroids, are anti-inflammatory in action. They are prescribed in patients who don't respond to NSAIDs or colchicines, especially elderly patients.

Preventing Attacks
Patients with renal disease, congestive heart failure and those taking diuretics are on high risk of getting another painful attack after sometime of the first attack. In these cases, NSAIDs must be given for one to two months to manage and prevent further attacks.

Chronic gout therapy
After treatment of acute gout, once all the symptoms are reduced, then starts an inter-critical period. It is the time when the decision to treat the patient with uricosuric drugs is being made. But that should be kept in mind that during inter-critical period, a sudden drop in uric acid level might aggravate acute gout attacks. To

avoid this condition patients are given colchicines prophylactically.

The aim is to facilitate uric acid excretion from the body, using uricosuric drugs or inhibiting its formation by giving xanthine oxidase inhibitors. Probenecid increase uric acid excretion by blocking tubular secretion of acids. It can cause gastrointestinal discomfort and should not be given to patients with nephrolithiasis. The starting dose is 250mg twice a day with a maximum daily dose of 3mg/d. Its use is ideal in those with 24hr urine uric acid excretion < 800mg. Xanthine oxidase inhibitor Allopurinol is well tolerated with mild side effects of gastric discomfort. Allopurinol, along with its metabolite oxypurinol, is effective in lowering uric acid levels and reducing tophus size. It's ideal for patients with urine uric acid levels > 8mg, renal insufficiency and tophaceous gout. The maintenance dose is 200-300mg/d. However, dose must be adjusted in renal insufficiency to avoid adverse effects. Some individuals may develop sensitivity in the first three months of therapy, known as Allopurinol hypersensitivity syndrome (AHS). Symptoms of sensitivity are allergic reactions and skin rash. In that case, medicine should be discontinued. Allopurinol is considered reliable in recurrent or tophaceous gout in comparison to uricosuric agents.

4) Disease States & Heredity

Hyperuricemia serves as a bridge to many serious health problems like high blood pressure and impaired kidney functions. Medicines must be given to manage high blood pressure and gout. Obesity, abnormally high or low level of lipids and high blood sugar level are other risk factors associated with gout. There has been good news for obese patients with studies now showing that lowering weight and following a healthy life style subsides symptoms of gout.

Rapid changes in the body contributes to metabolic syndrome, which is now considered a root cause of all these health problems including obesity, hypertension, high or low lipid levels, insulin resistance etc. The criterion for diagnosis is:
- Abdominal obesity (waist circumference of >102 cm in men and >88 cm in women),
- Hyper-triglyceridemia (high lipid levels).>150 mg/dl or 1.69 mmol/l,
- HDL (low high density lipoprotein cholesterol).<4omg/dl or 1.04 mmol/l in men and <50 mg/dl or 1.29mmol/l in women.

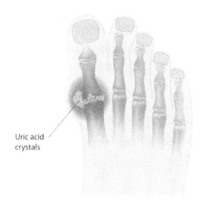

Uric acid
crystals

It's important to diagnose metabolic syndrome in gout patients, because the chances of cardiovascular diseases and diabetes mellitus in these patients are up to three and five times respectively. Mortality rates in patients with heart problems is higher with combined Hyperuricemia. Insulin resistance is also higher in gout patients as compared to healthy individuals. Theory suggests that it's a result of failure in renal uric acid secretion. Besides medicines there are certain dietary guidelines that must be followed to manage recurrent gout attacks.

Purine rich red meat including beef, lamb, pork, sausage, bologna, hot dog, chicken, turkey and vegetables including peas, lentils, mushrooms, cauliflower and oatmeal must be restricted in diet. Fructose in the diet must also be restricted, as fructose induced

Hyperuricemia is also observed in patients. It not only induces Hyperuricemia but also triggers high blood pressure. Sugar containing beverages increase serum uric acid levels irrespective of age, sex and gender.

So it's suggested that patients suffering from gout must avoid soft drinks to prevent increase in uric acid levels. People with abnormally high lipid levels must avoid alcohol, weight must be reduced by given fenofibrate to reduce their bad cholesterol and a healthy exercise routine must be followed to encourage HDL. High alcohol consumption is always associated with gout. But beer is supposed to be more harmful in triggering the gouty episodes since it contains guanosine, a type of purine that is converted to uric acid by action of enzymes. Many patients inform their physician that how certain foods and drinks trigger their pain.

Gout patients should follow four general rules to avoid pain attacks. Those patients who are overweight must reduce their weight by following a proper diet plan and exercise. Fasting blood lipid levels monitoring is necessary to make sure that hyperlipidemia is not the underlying cause behind it. If there are any symptoms of hyperlipidemia, then bad cholesterol (LDL) levels should be decreased and good cholesterol (HDL) levels should be increased by using appropriate medicines and diet. Patients must also be encouraged to have a quality diet and avoid red meat, beer and sugar containing beverages. High uric acid level is the precursor of kidney stones and gouty arthritis.

A study on SLC2A9 gene that transports fructose and glucose shows that urate transport is faster than glucose and fructose transport. It was revealed that urate transport gets faster in the presence of fructose moiety. So it was concluded that presence of fructose in a cell increases urate transport increasing uric acid concentration. Glucose and fructose binds with a different receptor protein. This study supports that high intake of fructose rich soft drinks and beverages increase overall body load of uric acid thereby causing Hyperuricemia and gouty arthritis.

High fructose intake not only triggers gout but also causes metabolic syndrome, which is the root cause of all illnesses. SLC2A9 is also found in chondrocytes. Cartilage transports urate because of this gene and cartilage is often considered the main site of urate crystals' deposition. Interleukin IL-1β, which is an inflammatory factor produced in gout, also facilitates the transport of glucose. GLUT9 transports uric acid faster than glucose or fructose transport. Being a transporter product of SLC2A9 gene it facilitates deposition of uric acid crystals in cartilage and joints causing inflammation and pain. IL-1β is a glucose transporter and this prompted researchers to determine its function in uric acid transportation via cartilage. Genetic changes influence uric acid levels beside biochemical changes in the body, however there are certain factors which suggest a rise in blood uric acid level is sometimes independent.

It's a very important factor in kidney functions impairment which not only creates kidney stones and inflammatory conditions like gouty arthritis, but proved to play an important role in developing heart problems and metabolic disorders. Proximal renal tubular cells of the kidney contain proteins, which play an important role in the transport of uric acid. The concentration gradient of transporter substances and transporter proteins such as URATI influences urate transport in kidney. URATI are found in proximal renal tubules of the kidney, which assist in reabsorption of uric acid.

Genetic changes in transport proteins present in the kidney influences urate transport. These transport proteins show single nucleotide polymorphisms, which also trigger the development of inflammation leading to Hyperuricemia gout.

One of the renal transport SLC2A9 gene product SNPs also show mutation which leads to Hyperuricemia and gout. A lot of research studies on genetic modifications on these transporter genes show that these genes exhibit a homozygous change in URATI (SLC22A12) gene, which builds the foundation for Hyperuricemia and gout. URATI is one of the key transporter proteins in renal function. So changes and genetic mutations in URATI make a lot of difference and cause Hyperuricemia because the reabsorption of urate in kidney is halted. Genetic changes in these transporter proteins are of two types naming hypouricimia and Hyperuricemia. In hypouricimia there is increased uric acid excretion, which causes failure of reabsorption by the kidney leading to hypouricimia, while when there is excessive reabsorption of uric acid by the kidney it leads to gout and Hyperuricemia.

Many other metabolites and chemicals react with URATI some times which either cause increase reabsorption or decreased excretion. Hyperuricemia and gout are also frequently associated with a term functional polymorphism besides genetic mutations in transporter protein mechanisms. The genes associated with glucose and fructose transport are GLUT9 or SLC2A9 are discussed earlier with their mechanism of fructose transport. Another study suggests that a G-family member (a family of receptors) ABCG2 gene is also a key factor which influences high serum uric acid levels in the body. It helps in the transport of uric acid from proximal tubules in the kidney, thereby decreasing uric acid concentration in cells. When polymorphism occurs in this gene, it reduces its ability to transport uric acid out of cell causing Hyperuricemia. Studies have shown that this genetic mutation is more common in males than females.

This mutation is also observed in China, where a study was conducted about prevalence while Asians also shows similar association. SLC17A1 is another gene, which is associated with serum uric acid transport in cell functions as uric acid secretor in the kidney. It's also associated with weight loss, and obese studies suggest that genetic mutation in this gene also contributes to gout.

The genetic changes in transporter proteins located in the proximal tubular region of the kidney are found to be responsible for Hyperuricemia and gout, and shows the correlation of genetic mutation with gout. Kidneys, which play a vital role in uric acid transport, are a great platform to study and design new medicines for gout. The study of all the genes susceptible to genetic mutation provides a medium to better understanding of the risk and prevalence in different populations and people.

5) Genetic Abnormalities

Inherited defects which lead to Hyperuricemia and gout are glucose-6-phosphatase (G6PT) deficiency, hypoxanthine-guanine phosphoribosyl-transferase (HGPRT) deficiency, and elevated 5'-phosphoribosyl-1'-pyrophosphate synthetase (PRPP). Deficiency in glucose-6-phosphatase results in type I glycogen storage disease.

Juvenile gout also known as Lesch–Nyhan syndrome (LNS) affects more exclusively male. It's characterized by excess uric acid levels with neurological abnormalities. Deficiency of enzyme hypoxanthine-guanine phosphoribosylatransferase (HGPRT) due to mutation in HGPRT gene cause juvenile gout. This deficiency causes an imbalance of uric acid in the body, causing Hyperuricemia. The genes which are responsible for uric acid transportation are SLC2A9 (GLUT9) and ABCG2.

Studies have shown that these genes have a strong influence on urate concentration and development of gout. Unfortunately, this genetic control on inflammation is not understood yet, as there is not much information available. This encoded protein SLC2A9 also nourishes chondrocytes in cartilages. Transporter proteins such as URATI mediates urate reabsorption from proximal renal tubules in the kidney. Mutation in these proteins plays an important role in developing Hyperuricemia and gout.

Individuals suffering from Hyperuricemia and gout develop a homozygous mutation in URATI. Genome wide association studies (GWAS) conclude that SLC2A9 and ABCG2 have a strong relation with increased serum urate levels and gout. Studies suggest a strong correlation of genetic control on serum urate levels but not on coronary heart disease and blood pressure. Furthermore, the genetic mutations which are responsible for development of Hyperuricemia and gout have no association with other health problems related to it.

Chapter 3: Main Stages of Gout Disorder

It is best understood by dividing it into four stages. Gout proceeds in four stages. Theses stages are as follows:
1) - Asymptomatic Hyperuricemia
2) - Acute gouty arthritis
3) - Inter-critical period
4) - Advanced or chronic tophaceous gout.

1) Stage # 1: Asymptomatic Hyperuricemia

It is a stage that is prior to the first attack of gout and as the name implies it has no symptoms. Although, there is a higher concentration of uric acid in blood, still treatment is not required and is unnecessary at this stage.

2) Stage # 2: Acute Attacks

Acute attacks are usually characterized by the following conditions;
- Sudden onset of pain especially at night,
- Swelling, warmth and redness of joint,
- Chills,
- Tachycardia,
- Malaise,
- Fever,
- Skin becomes red or purplish.

These conditions occur because of deposition of uric acid crystals in joints. These uric acid crystals initiate inflammation and pain around the joint ,which is called bursitis. Acute gout usually attacks the first metatarsophalangeal joint (the big toe) and it is called podagra. Nonetheless, it can also affect other joints as well including fingers, wrist, elbow, knee, ankle and instep. The pain attack is very severe and usually happens at night and lasts up to two weeks if left untreated. When there is an episode of a second attack, it spreads pain in other joints as well.

Joints Effected By Gout:

Mono-articular Gout: when only one joint is effected it is called mono-articular gout. Big toes are the most effected joint in first attacks. But other locations like the knee or ankle can also be affected. It mostly affects middle-aged people.

Polyarticular Gout: As the name implies, it affects multiple joints. Older people are more at risk of poly-articular gout. Foot, wrist, elbow, ankle, knee and hand are most affected. Pain radiates in one side of body, usually the legs and feet. Pain starts slowly and the intervals between attacks are longer. They suffer from fever, loss of appetite and overall bad health. When the first symptoms appear, then the pain goes to peak in 24-48 hours and subsides after 5-7 days if left untreated. These attacks can last up to hours to several weeks. Symptoms are subsided after a few hours but the presence of crystals is a sign of more future attacks.

The main purpose of therapy is to sink down or precipitate pain and improve quality of life. If it is not treated in early stages sings of pain disappear to several weeks. Many anti-inflammatory drugs are available to treat acute gout which includes NSAIDs, colchicine, and glucocorticoids.

Following measures should be taken to treat acute gout:

a) After the first attack of pain it is ideal to start the treatment as soon as possible. Symptoms should begin to sink down and precipitate as the treatment progresses. Treatment should be started with the recommended dose of anti-inflammatory medicine. If an attack begins during treatment, the dose must be reduced to half to achieve desired results.

b) Once the symptoms of the pain are subsided completely, then treatment can be stopped. But in case of oral glucocorticoids, slight tapering is required to prevent a recurrent attack.

c) Treatment period can range from a day to several weeks. Some patients might only need five to seven days if treatment is started right on-time within 12hours of first attack.

d) During the initial stage of acute attack drugs used to lower uric acid are not beneficial. But if patient is already receiving these medicines, then they must be continued to prevent another attack.

e) Treatment guidelines for both patients are same.

f) Treatment recommendations for patients with or without tophi are almost similar.

g) Presence of tophi is an indication of long-term treatment plan to prevent chronic gouty arthritis.

h) In patients who have other medical illnesses and receiving other therapies, dose must be adjusted accordingly, as it might affect the dugs effectiveness.

i) Care must be taken if patients have one of the following conditions:
- Renal function
- Heart problems
- Gastrointestinal diseases
- Drug Allergy
- Diabetes

j) Some adjunctive measures are icing of effected joint and taking analgesic medications.

Medicines are select according to the current health and treatment the patient is already receiving. Treatment is started with an oral anti-inflammatory medicine to those who can take oral medicines. Those who can take oral medicines but NSAIDs are fatal to their health because of an illness such as chronic kidney disease, peptic ulcer or history of NSAIDs intolerance, are given colchicine. Then those patients who can't take both NSAIDs and colchicine are given intra-articular, oral or parenteral steroids/glucocorticoids.

The first line agents are NSAIDs, as they don't have much contraindication and are well tolerated. As initial therapy, a potent NSAID such as naproxen 500mg twice daily or Indomethacin 50mg is given thrice a day. After the symptoms are reduced, this NSAID therapy can be ceased after three days. Duration of treatment with NSAIDs is 5-7 days depending on the condition. NSAIDs therapy is of short duration in patients where treatment begun just after the first attack. Aspirin is not prescribed for the treatment of gouty arthritis.

If patient can't tolerate NSAIDs then a low dose of oral colchicine 1.5 to 1.8mg in two or three divided doses in 24 hours is given. However, intravenous administration of colchicines is contraindicated. Patients who can't take oral medicines are given oral glucocorticoid injections. Triamcinolone acetonide 40mg can be prescribed for a large joint (knee), and 30mg for medium joint (wrist, ankle, and elbow) or methylprednisolone acetate in equivalent doses.

Patients who can't take oral NSAIDs or colchicines neither injection of glucocorticoid are given oral steroids such as prednisone 30-50mg once daily or an equivalent till pain is gone. Patients with extreme pain and flares required 10-14 days to overcome the pain.
Intravenous glucocorticoid is suggested in patients with intolerance to oral medicines. Methylprednisolone 20mg is given twice daily. It's reduced to half when improvements start and

adjusted to 4mg twice daily for five days. Intramuscular injection can also be used.

Patients who are unresponsiveness to other therapies can be given interleukin inhibitors such as canakinumab or anakinra.

3) Stage # 3: Inter-critical Periods

The period between attacks is defined as inter-critical period. After first attack, symptoms subside for a period of time. Unfortunately, if gout is left untreated it may reoccur with extreme pain. Usually this phase is asymptomatic and can last from months to years.

4) Stage # 4: Advanced Gout

After many years, gout develops in chronic tophaceous gout. Studies suggest that it takes almost 10 years to the damage until tophi is formed. Solid crystals of uric acid are formed in joints, cartilage, bones and hands. These nodule-like appearance are called crab eyes.

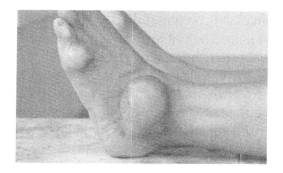

Women are at more risk of developing tophi. When gout is not treated well then the period between attacks gets shorter and pain becomes intense. Tophi can be formed in the helix of ear, forearms, elbow, knee, hands and feet.
Tophi are painless but they produce stiffness in the effected area.

After complete treatment tophi dissolve and disappear. Surgical interventions are required when tophi interfere with the functions of tendons or cause skin necrosis or ulceration and when tophi cause compression on nerves. As uric acid crystals are bacteriostatic there is mild infection. Tophi can impair circulation in tissue. General anesthesia is recommended in surgical procedures. There is a life-long treatment for gout. So a definite diagnosis must be made on time. It may be very easy to diagnose gout when a patient has a clear situation of disease but joints could also get inflamed in two or more possible causes. So the first step is to diagnose which joint is affected. Physical examination and medical history supports the presence of gout. If it appears in the big toe then it is most likely to be gouty arthritis.

Duration of pain attacks and swelling are also key factors. Symptoms which appear after weeks indicate other problem than gout. For diagnosis of gout, synovial fluid examination is considered an accurate method. Synovium is filled with a lubricating fluid called synovial fluid. Joints are surrounded by this membrane, which protects it from sheer damage.

This fluid not only supports joints but also provides essential nourishment and oxygen to cartilage, hence protecting bones in multiple ways. This examination is even useful between inter-critical periods to diagnose gout. The whole procedure is called arthrocentesis in which fluid is drawn from the effected joint using a needle attached to a syringe. Then this sample is sent to the laboratory for further examination. If it indicates presence of monosodium crystals in the fluid, it is possibly gout. This process somehow also reduces the inflammation and pressure build around the joint, easing pain. However, a blood test can also be performed to measure uric acid levels in blood.

A blood test is often inaccurate, because the level of uric acid seems to rise during an attack and falls after the pain subsides. So it's better to take a blood test right after an attack.

Chapter 4: Purine Biochemistry

Overview: This whole phenomenon of purine metabolism represents a natural process, which breaks different components in cells and tissues. In this chapter we will explore the mechanisms and functions of specific purine bases and their role in triggering gout.

1) Structure

Purine can be best described as a group of natural substances found in all cells of our body and in many foods as well. They are the most commonly occurring nitrogenous compounds in nature. Then a question pops up in mind of 'what is the purpose of their abundance in nature?' The answer is they are the building blocks of our genes. However their chemical structure is composed of a pyrimidine ring attached to an imidazole ring.

Together purine and pyrimidine make deoxyribonucleic acid (DNA) and ribonucleic acid (RNA). Two naturally occurring purines include adenine and guanine. These purine bases form hydrogen bonds with pyrimidines thymine and cytosine in DNA. Purine bases are composed of 6 membered and 5 membered nitrogen rings in the system. While pyrimidine has a 6 membered ring structure with two nitrogens and four carbons in the ring system. Although they both have 6 membered rings, they are not the same metabolically. A sugar moiety along with a purine or pyrimidine forms a nucleoside. Further attachment of a phosphate group with this sugar part makes a nucleotide.

Purine bases occur in the form of nucleosides, nucleotides and nucleic acid in the body. Purines and their derivatives along with uric acid were first discovered by Emil Fischer. As discussed earlier, purine ring is formed by a combination of 4 and 5 carbon atoms of pyrimidine and imidazole ring. The chemical name of this compound is 7(9)-H-imidazole (4, 5-d) pyrimidine (fig 6.1). Fischer also isolated adenine but it was Kossel in 1885 that isolated adenine from beef pancreas along with guanine and confirmed it as a part of DNA. Then, later on, other constituents like thymine, cytosine and uracil were also isolated by his team. The discovery of hypoxanthine and xanthine adds a milestone in the study of gout and related diseases. Allopurinol, a hypoxanthine analog, is of significant importance in study of gout.

There is a change in carbon at position no 8 and nitrogen in position no 7 besides the presence of a hydroxyl group in position 6 in the ring. It's an important agent in lowering serum uric acid levels. 6 mercaptopurine is another compound of significant importance (fig.6.3). This compound is obtained by reacting hypoxanthine with phosphorus pentasulfide.

This compound has anti-cancer and antitumor activities. But the sulfhydryl group of mercaptopurine undergoes oxidation. To address this problem, azathioprine was formulated, which is a mercaptopurine analog. It's a potent immunosuppressive agent.

2) Nucleic Acid Degradation

Our body produces uric acid when purines are broken down in the body. To get a deeper understanding of gout and what the external and internal factors that trigger such a painful episodes of inflammation are, we must understand and consider all the factors responsible for uric acid accumulation in the body.

The excess of uric acid in body is either due to a purine rich diet, tissue turnover or purine metabolism. Purine metabolites after passing through catabolism are converted into uric acid by different enzymes; enzyme endonuclease hydrolyzes DNA and RNA. It breaks chemical bonds present between polynucleotide chains. These nucleotides have a purine base attached with ribose or deoxyribose phosphate. Ribose nucleotides undergo guanylic pathway. Adenylate deaminase enzyme deaminates adenylic acid and reduces it to inosinic acid. Later on, inosinic acid and guanylic acid are further hydrolyzed by phosphomonoesterases. This enzyme further breaks these metabolites into nucleosides which are cleaved by another enzyme nucleoside phosphorylases and form the purine bases guanine and hypoxanthine.

The process that represent the breaking of cells and tissues in the body is termed as tissue turnover i.e. the process by which new cells are formed. When the cells in our body die i.e. programmed cell death, the purine in them also destroys. So as a result, uric acid is formed due to purine breakdown. This buildup of uric acid leads to accumulation of uric acid crystals in joints, tendons and kidneys; causing gout.

3) De Novo Synthesis of Purine Nucleotides.

De Novo purine nucleotide synthesis occurs in the liver. In this pathway, purines and uric acid are synthesized. Therefore De Novo synthesis is crucial in understanding the precursors and pathway, which triggers gout. Purine nucleotide is formed from contribution of 4, 5 carbons and 7 nitrogen of glycine, amino nitrogen of aspartate, 3 and 9 nitrogen atoms from amide of glutamine, carbon dioxide, 1 nitrogen atom from aspartic acid and ribose 5-Phosphate.

a) Synthesis of 5-phosphoribosyl-1-pyrophosphate (PRPP):
Described as an activated pentose PRPP actively participates in the formation of nucleotides i.e. purine and pyrimidines. Adenosine tri phosphate (ATP) and ribose 5-phosphate synthesize PRPP. This reaction is catalyzed by an enzyme PRPP synthetase. Inorganic phosphate activates this enzyme.

b) Synthesis of 5'-phosphoribosylamine:
PRPP and glutamine synthesize 5'-phosphoribosylamine. The pyrophosphate group attached with carbon 1 of PRPP is replaced by amide group of glutamine. AMP and GMP, which are the end products of this pathway, inhibit the enzyme phosphoribosyl

pyrophosphate amidotransferase. In purine nucleotide biosynthesis this step is called the committed step. The intracellular concentration of PRPP present in the cell controls the rate of reaction. Hence the concentration of PRPP effects and controls the rate of reaction.

c) Synthesis of inosine monophosphate:
In the third nitrogen of amino group a formyl group is attached. Tetrahydrofolic acid is required in this step which forms an intermediate 5- formamido- 4- imidazole- carboxamide- ribotide. The ring closure at nitrogen 1 and carbon 2 forms inosine, monophosphate (IMP) or inosinic acid, which is also called the parent nucleotide. It requires ATP as energy source.

4) AMP & GMP

The conversion of IMP to AMP and GMP is a two-step process which requires a lot of energy. Guanosine triphosphate is an energy source for the formation of AMP, while adenosine triphosphate is required for GMP. The end products formed at the end of each pathway inhibits the first reaction in each pathway. The logic behind this inhibition has a sole purpose of diverting IMP to form purine compounds in the end, thereby inhibiting excess production of uric acid. The presence of AMP and GMP is sufficient enough to inhibit the purine synthesis at the amidotransferase step.

5) Salvage Pathway For Purines

The parent purine base inosinic acid consumes 6 ATP molecules in de novo purine pathway. These purine bases are excreted in urine if the salvage pathway was not there. This process of reutilization preserves these purine bases. This process is catalyzed by an enzyme phosphoribosyl transferases (PRT). It influences the addition of 5-phosphate in base to form a nucleotide.

Base + PRPP = Base-ribose-phosphate (BMP) + PPi
BMP= Base monophosphate

Conversion of purine bases to nucleotides

Two enzymes, namely adenine phosphoribosyltransferase
(APRT) and hypoxanthine-guanine phosphoribosyltransferase
(HGPRT), are important in this process. They both utilize PRPP
from ribose 5-phosphate.

Lesch- Nyhan Syndrome:
The deficiency of HGPRT causes Lesch-Nyhan syndrome. Due to
deficiency of this enzyme, salvaging of hypoxanthine and guanine
is halted. Due to which the end product of uric acid is formed in
excess quantity in body. It also causes an increase in PRPP levels,
thereby decreasing IMP and GMP levels in the body. Due to this
imbalance, the committed step in purine synthesis is also halted
and there are increased amounts of substrates and decreased
inhibitors. This condition facilitates degradation of purine and
related compounds leading to excess formation of uric acid. It's
an inherited disorder in which patient suffers from
Hyperuricemia, accumulation of uric acid crystals in the kidney
causing urolithiasis and accumulation of uric acid in joints and
tissues causing gout.

Degradation of Purine Nucleotides

Dietary nucleic acids are broken down in the small intestine
where it's converted to nucleotides by enzymatic action. Many
nucleosides, along with free bases, are produced and uric acid
being the end product of the reaction.

a) Degradation of dietary nucleic acids in small intestine
Dietary RNA and DNA are hydrolyzed to oligonucleotides by
two enzymes; ribonucleases and deoxyribonucleases. Then, the
pancreatic enzyme phosphodiesterase hydrolyze them to 3' and 5'
mononucleotides. Then their phosphate group is reduced to

nucleosides and free bases. These dietary purines are converted to uric acid in the intestine and then excreted in the urine.

b) Formation of Uric acid

As discussed earlier, AMP is converted into IMP. Then IMP and GMP are converted into nucleosides inosine and guanosine by an enzyme 5'-nucleotidase. These are further converted into hypoxanthine and guanine by purine nucleoside phosphorylase. Amino group is removed from guanine to form xanthine. xanthine oxidase enzyme oxidize hypoxanthine to form uric acid.

Chapter 5: Getting The Right Diagnosis

As discussed earlier, the gout can be very confusing with other injuries and arthritis. So, it's very important to make the right diagnosis at the right time. Gout treatment can be life-long and needs a proper care and change in lifestyle. Injuries and trauma of the toe or any other joint can be confused with gout, so care must be taken in making the right decision. Many patients with gout also have hypertension and impaired kidney functions, therefore a proper medical examination of cardiac and kidney functions is necessary. Some of the baseline tests crucial in diagnosing of gout are discussed below.

1) Synovial Fluid Diagnosis

The viscous fluid in the cavities of the synovial joints is termed as synovial fluid. This fluid is responsible to reduce friction between joints during movement. Presence of mono sodium urate crystals in synovial fluids serves as an identification marker for the diagnosis of gout. A Sample is collected by drawing the fluid from the affected joint with the help of a needle. Care must be taken while drawing the fluid and must be done by an expert. Samples should be kept and handle with care as their solubility are affected by temperature and pH. So examination must be performed quickly right after aspiration from inflamed joint. Microscopic examination reveals the presence of urate crystals in joints.

The two identification tests for inflamed joints and gouty arthritis include arthrocentesis and synovial fluid analysis. In case of arthritis, synovial fluid culture and sensitivity tests are performed. If the sample examination shows a white blood cell count more than 100,000 cells/mm^3, surely it's a sign of infection in joints.

The chances of sepsis are less when the count appears to be less than 50,000 cells/mm³. Patients who underwent organ transplant and are immune-compromised usually have a low neutrophil count in sepsis and inflammation.

The presence of uric acid crystals in the sample are proof of gout in patients. However there are many infections, which also increase the occurrence of uric acid crystals in the body.

Arthrocentesis
This procedure is used for large and complex joints like the ankle, knee and wrist. Aspiration is quite difficult for small joints like hip, shoulder and finger. Joint aspirations must be performed by an experienced clinician and care must be taken during the procedure. The effected place is cleaned with soap and water. Alcohol and iodine are used to swab the place. In case of any allergy only alcohol is used instead of iodine.

Anesthetic agents like Xylocaine and ethyl chloride spray are used for anesthesia. Xylocaine must be used in accurate measures as increased anesthesia can result in altered results. 25 gauge sized needles can be used to give Xylocaine. Aspiration needles' size ranges from 16-18. To prevent synovial fluid from clotting, an anticoagulant sodium heparin is used. Syringe is wet with sodium heparin to prevent clotting. Alternate solutions are sodium citrate and ethylene diaminetetra acetic acid (EDTA). Whereas solutions of oxalate and lithium heparin must not be used because these solutions are also crystal based and might create confusion in distinguishing uric acid crystals. Surgical gloves can also contaminate the synovial fluid with talc so care must be taken while handling the sample. 1-5 ml of fluid is collected for examination.

This process also decreases swelling in the joint by reducing pressure on it. For that purpose, a hub is attached to the syringe for exchange of fluids. Lateral and medial sites are considered ideal for knee aspirations and fluid is pushed towards the needle by pushing the opposite side of the needle. In case of gonococcal infections where the pus site is complex lateral and medial sites are utilized. The aspiration site for wrist is radiocarpal joint. The ankle is aspirated from the anterior side and shoulder is aspirated using anterior or posterior positions.

The dorsolateral approach is utilized for finger joints. Now many books and CD's are available which easily guide a clinician to perform aspiration. Sterilization should be of prime concern and care must be taken while performing aspirations to avoid complications. If not properly done, aspiration technique could cause infections, pain and hemarthroses. Local anesthetic agents eliminate chances of pain and discomfort during the procedure. One of the common effects of this procedure is fainting, so it is necessary that the patient must have an attendant to handle any emergency. Patients with bleeding disorders must be treated prior to their aspiration to avoid any complication.

It is very rare to have infections after aspiration if properly performed. Skin must be examined before performing aspiration and this procedure should not be continued if there are cuts or lesions. Skin lesions contain infectious organisms, which might enter during aspiration and can cause sepsis.

Studies reveal that the reasons contributing to the failure of aspiration technique are the thickness of synovial fluid, lipoma arborescens or adipose tissues. When fat comes along with synovial fluid it results in lipoma arborescens. Knee aspirations must be performed from the lateral side for best results. It is believed that the sample examination must be performed quickly after aspiration because temperature changes the solubility of samples and effects end results.

After 24hrs, white blood cell count decreases by about 1,000-4,000 cells/mm^3 and crystals are difficult to recognize. Many artifactual crystals are also formed in synovial fluid, which affects the examination. Uric acid crystals remain in sample for almost 8 weeks but they are very difficult to recognize and small in size.

Synovial fluid culture
Gout and septic arthritis are the main factors responsible for inflammation and synovitis. There are four diagnostic tests performed for diagnosis of gout. These tests are culture and sensitivity of fluid, synovial fluid smears for gram stain and blood cell count including white blood cell differential count, total white blood cell count and wet preparations. These cultures may not be 100% accurate.

However, the laboratory environment must be sterilize and hygienic to minimize chances of infection. Elderly patients and children are more likely to develop infections. Medical ailments such as prosthetic joints, diabetes mellitus, rheumatoid arthritis, sickle cell disease and chronic liver diseases are more likely to increase complications in patients. Synovial fluid specimens are very sensitive and prone to temperature. If the test is performed late there are very less chances of a positive culture.

Anerobic bacteria are rarely responsible for joint inflammations but unhygienic clinical conditions can cause such complications. However there are a lot of factors, which are responsible for increasing the risks of anerobic infections including immunocompromised patient, trauma due to syringe and prosthetic joints. If such infection occurs then culture test for the anaerobe is performed.

Synovial fluid gram stain
Synovial fluid is of utmost importance in determining the signs of infectious organisms. Right after that, antibiotic therapy is started for treatment. These cultures provide 50-70% result and one can easily differentiate among gram positive and gram negative bacteria. But the drawback of gram stains are they can't identify between staphylococcus and streptococcus infections. They also can't differentiate between infectious arthritis and gout.

The slides and apparatus used in examination must be clean to get accurate results. A good way to sterilize cover slips and slides is application of acetone. After examination of gram stain results, antibiotic therapy must be initiated to treat infection.

Synovial fluid white blood cell count

A white blood cell count of 2,000 cells/mm^3 is considered normal in synovial fluid. By contrary, some inflammatory conditions like systemic lupus erythematosus, arthritis, sclerosis and synovitis show this count. Synovial fluid shows non-unflammatory white blood cell count in other inflammatory conditions as well as sickle cell disease, gland disorders and hyperlipoproteinemia. Studies also reveal that immune-compromised patients also have low white blood cell count in Hyperuricemia and gout.

Clinical findings reveal a total white blood cell count of 50,000-100,000 cells/mm3 in infection related arthritis and crystal induced arthritis. Lot of research and studies show the importance of white blood cell count and neutrophil count in synovial fluid. It serves as an identification tool to distinguish between the inflammatory and non-inflammatory state of a joint. Levels of other chemical compounds such as protein, glucoseand lactic acid dehydrogenase are equally important but levels of white blood cells and neutrophils serve as a standard identification marker for inflammations as a result of infection and gout.

They are considered as critical criteria for diagnosis of gout. People who suffer from systemic sclerosis, systemic lupus erythematosus and tissue disorders develop more complications with gout. Diagnosis must be made clearly to avoid confusion between tissue disorder and gout. Samples of synovial fluid must be examined under critical conditions to make the right diagnosis. We know that gout can make the situation worse for patients already suffering from increased uric acid levels and lupus.

There was a myth that gout does not affect the black population much compared to others but after surveys it was revealed that alcohol intake, kidney problems and high blood pressure and gout are commonly present in black as well. Formerly known as the disease of kings it now affects almost all populations in the world because of the lack of a healthy life style.

Most of the times joint inflammation occurs due to bacterial infections, which are confused with other medical problems such as connective tissue disorders. Untill now, many attempts are made to formulate diagnostic tests and criteria for correct diagnosis of disease. Many studies and research results show that the bacterial infections account for most of the inflammatory conditions in the body including auto immune disorders, rheumatoid arthritis and joint disease of the vertebral column. Now the situation relies on the identification inflammatory markers, which are used as a standard to identify septic arthritis,

Hyperuricemia and gout. Secondly, the criteria of observing markers, which do not appear in the result, are also sometimes used to eliminate confusions in making diagnosis. Many laboratory results have shown normal white blood cell count in different inflammatory conditions, which is quite misleading. It's very important to distinguish between septic arthritis and gout. Sometimes, it is very difficult to distinguish among them.

Most of the time, these tests are unable to give accurate results. Although DNA amplification of samples can give appropriate results in identification between bacterial infection induced inflammation and crystal induced inflammation. This technique sometimes helps in identifying the underlying disease and suspected organism. There is still a long way to go, as sometimes bacterial DNA analysis in samples is not sufficient enough to provide accurate results for diagnosis. There is a lot of data and an in depth study is required for the structure and chemical properties of bacteria causing septic arthritis.

Bacterial DNA must be analyzed in synovial fluid for identification of suspected organisms. To make the long story short, synovial fluid, its culture test and examination serves as an important tool for diagnosing many joint disorders and their root causes. The underlying issues can be addressed if a correct diagnosis is made.

When a patient comes up with a swollen joint, immediate action must be taken and aspiration and examination of organisms and compounds present in the sample are a crucial step. There are many exceptions to the rules and criteria of the examination.

The differential count of the sample showing 90% neutrophil and 50,000-100,000 cells/mm^3 shows the presence of septic or gouty arthritis in the body. Slides must be prepared with extreme caution and use of an appropriate polarized microscope is of great help in identifying uric acid crystals and gout.

2) Tophi Sampling Diagnosis

Mono sodium urate crystals often deposit in the form of a mass called tophi. It is an indicator of abnormally high levels of uric acid in the body. Tophus is the final warning for the body for proper treatment, as studies suggests that people who develop tophi already have attacks of gout. It's in the form of white chalky nodules. They are visible and can be seen around joints and pinna of ear. These nodules are also termed as gout nodules and gout pearls. These tophi are very painful and cause difficulty in movement. Imaging studies which are performed for the identification of intra articular tophi are difficult.

Tophi are more easily diagnosed when calcified. They are not visible on plain radiographs. Cross sectional imaging with CT or MRI are performed for large and complex joints, for example the knee. It helps in determining the nature and type of nodules that form tophi. They are diagnostic tools for chronic tophaceous gout. It could be a better diagnostic option than radiography for determining presence of tophi and erosions. Ultrasonography is also a useful tool besides cross sectional diagnosis. A drop of fluid is placed on a slide and observed under polarizing microscope. Under the microscope, uric acid appears in the form of yellow or blue needle-like structures.

Tophi with periarticular masses are rare and must not be confused with neoplasms. Many urate crystals combine and form a mass, which contain chalky white amorphous material. Microscopic examination of a sample shows the presence of stacks of needle shaped crystals along with inflammatory markers. Polarized microscopes confirm the presence of uric acid crystals. Increase in serum uric acid levels further confirms the presence of gout and this mass is identified as gouty tophi. Tophi are attached with a proteinaceous covering and contain foreign giant cells and macrophages. Periarticular and subcutaneous tissues are mostly affected by tophi. It's formed near knee, forearm, Achilles tendon and the helix of the ear.

Usually, it can affect any joint of the body. But these sites are the most common sites for tophi formation the reason is these sites are considered cooler parts of the body. Determination of uric acid levels in serum is of not much help. Many alcoholics have lower serum uric acid levels similar to diabetic patients who also have normal or lower serum uric acid levels because of increased glucose levels wiping of uric acid rapidly from the body. Slides of the samples must be handled and prepared with extreme care as during the preparation many monosodium urate crystals destroy. But use of proper solvents and alcohol helps in fixing the smears. Under examining in polarized light they reveal the presence of crystals. Such a crystalline tophi, is usually diagnosed for tumoral calcinosis and pseudo-gout and should not be mixed and confused with neoplasms. Both the conditions are characterized by tissue calcification. It is diagnosed by radiology.

The difference between the yield of gouty tophi and tumoral calcinosis and pseudo-gout is the presence of thick basophilic calcified substances in the sample. Whereas, the sample of gout shows needle like crystals of mono sodium urate (MSU)).

Another difference is that tumoral calcinosis tophi contains powder like amorphous aspirate which are non crystalline in structure. In pseudo-gout the crystals are rhomboid or needle shaped and are much smaller in size as compared to MSU crystals which are much bigger in size. Thus, fine needle aspiration cytology (FNAC) helps in the diagnosis and treatment of gout at the right time.

3) Blood Test For Uric Acid Level

It helps in determining levels of uric acid in the body. Patients undergoing chemotherapy or radiation treatment for cancer also need to check their uric acid levels, as these treatments increase the risk of increased uric acid. High levels of uric acid in the blood are a sign of Hyperuricemia, which is due to overproduction and under excretion of uric acid from body.

However, the low levels of uric acid are often linked with kidney or liver diseases. Some people have abnormally high levels of uric acid in the blood without any signs of disease, which is asymptomatic Hyperuricemia. Blood samples should be collected for the diagnosis of gout. Many medications such as ibuprofen, aspirin, high levels of vitamin c and alcohol interact with uric acid results. So it's required to check if the patient is taking any over the counter or prescription drug to avoid any possible interaction. The patient needs to fast and must refrain from eating and drinking for four hours before the test. This test is called venipuncture.

The area is sterilized with an antiseptic solution then an elastic band is tied up to fill the veins with blood. The doctor will draw blood from the vein of the inner elbow or back of the hand. The normal range of uric acid ranges between 3.5-7.2 mg of uric acid per deciliter of blood. Low levels are more uncommon than high levels. High levels suggest diabetes and gout.

Blood tests are safe, but the patient might feel pain at the site, bleeding, fainting or lightheadedness, hematoma or bruising. However, a blood test is not a foolproof method for the identification of gout. As blood uric acid levels rise and fall during the painful episodes of the attack. An inter-critical period can be utilized and the physician must wait after an attack. If this test does not help to diagnose gout then another possible test is synovial fluid test.

4) Urine Test

Urine analysis is recommended if the doctor suspects high levels of uric acid. The test is done to check uric acid levels and kidney stones. Make sure the patient is not taking any medication or supplement which can alter the results.

A 24 hour urine sample is collected and normally you would fast of four hours before the test is required. It is not the first thing collected in the morning first the patient need to empty bladder completely in morning note the time then urine is collected every time when its urge for bathroom over 24 hour period. The container is capped and sealed and placed in the refrigerator and sent to laboratory for urine analysis. A healthy adult normally loses 500-600mg of uric acid in urine every 24 hours. More than 800 mg per day is considered a high level and needs consideration. If there are high levels of uric acid in the urine then enzyme tests are performed to confirm the presence of the disease. Another possible complication could be kidney stones.

5) HLA - Tissue Typing Test

The genome wide association studies (GWAS) reveal that many genes which are responsible to transport uric acid are linked with renal urate transport. So, the renal decrease renal urate excretion accounts for gout in 90% of patients. The genes which are found in renal proximal tubules are termed as uric acid transportasome.

This group includes glucose transporter type 9 (GLUT9) also called SLC2A9, urate anion transporter 1(URATI) also called as SLC22A12 and ATP binding ABCG2.

The test for urate associated genes lacks utility and is found to be very limited because serum uric acid levels are enough to predict gout. The human leukocyte antigen (HLA) makes a group of proteins which are located on the surface of white blood cells. Our immune system uses these HLA to identify between self and non self proteins made by virus and bacteria. HLA is a version of major histocompatibility complex (HMC).

Humans have three MHC genes HLA-A, HLA -B and HLA-C. These genes are involved in protection of the immune system and inflammation. These genes have a lot of variations and around 100 medical conditions are related to mutations in these genes. Many inflammatory disorders are associated with HLA-B gene. HLA-B27 is a blood test, which identifies the protein located in white blood cells.

This particular gene can cause immune system dysfunction and its presence on white blood cells causes the immune system to attack normal healthy white blood cells, which results in autoimmune diseases. This test is performed when there are symptoms of joint pain and inflammation, stiffness in the neck, spine or chest and inflammation of the eye. The test is set on a standard blood draw performed by an expert nurse, clinician or technician. Blood is drawn from arm using a needle and sample is sent to a laboratory for examination.

No special preparation is required and the patient should be asked to stop taking any medicine, which can alter the results. This test has minimum risks and the patient may experience lightheadedness, or infection at the site, excessive bleeding or fainting. If the test is positive it may be indicative of an auto immune disorder but final diagnosis is based on the results of all blood tests and examinations and symptoms.

6) Medical Conditions Similar To Gout

a) Juvenile arthritis
Children of age 16 or younger suffer from this arthritis. No particular test for its diagnosis is helpful. It affects bone development in children. Painful episodes last for six weeks in the patient.

b) Ankylosing spondylitis
It's a very painful inflammation of the spine where the bones grow together. This is due to the presence of HLA-B27 gene on white blood cells.

c) System lupus erythematous
This inflammatory disorder is characterized by swelling of joints, tendons, connective tissues and organs including heart, lung, kidney and skin.

Chapter 6: Hyperuricemia

1) What is Hyperuricemia?

Being an antioxidant in nature uric acid's primary role is detoxification of the body. In humans, uric acid is the end product of purine metabolism. Our body gets rid of excessive purine nucleosides by a break down in the liver and excreting them from the kidneys. In mammals, uric acid is formed during purine metabolism, which is converted to allantoin by the action of an enzyme uricase.

Allantoin is a soluble compound, which is excreted from body later on. Unfortunately, after genetic mutations humans and some primates lack uricase enzyme. The two important organs which play an important role in uric acid excretion are liver and kidney. The liver synthesizes uric acid as formed by the degradation of purines. Dysfunctional kidney can also contributes to excessive uric acid levels in blood. A mutation in the urate transport system of the kidney causes failure to excrete uric acid from the body thereby causing increased levels of uric acid in the blood.

It's always thought of as an end product of purine metabolism but our body needs to maintain a healthy balance of it in small proportions. It is more likely because of its role as an antioxidant in the body. It neutralizes 50% of harmful toxins or free radicals in the blood stream. Humans and primates preserve uric acid due to slow filtration and lack of uricase enzyme. But this scenario in return can powerfully increase antioxidant function of the blood.

This uric acid in normal levels protects our brain from damage. Therefore low levels of uric acid are also associated with neurological problems such as multiple sclerosis, Huntington's, Parkinson's and Alzheimer's.

The normal range of uric acid in blood is 8.6mg/dl in men and 7.1mg/dl in women. Many laboratories and clinical teams use different standard limits.

Hyperuricemia is a precursor of gout and initiates a series of painful episodes, although many patients suffer from asymptomatic Hyperuricemia and do not develop any symptoms. Hyperuricemia is the risk factor for gout. In its absence, gout does not occur. Uric acid levels vary among different populations and there are many factors that influence it. Asymptomatic Hyperuricemia is a risk factor for development of other medical conditions in the body. It serves as a gateway to more complications, thereby reducing the quality of life.

As patients with asymptomatic Hyperuricemia never experience an attack ultrasounds are found to be helpful in diagnosis. These studies have shown inflammation and swelling around the joints. However. as the levels of uric acid increase in body, risk of gout also increases. When the blood uric acid level starts rising and not excreting from the body, monosodium urate crystals start accumulating in cartilage and soft tissues causing redness, pain and inflammation.

These crystals can stay in the body without causing pain. Two things can happen with uric acid crystals; either they enter the circulation again or shed by tissue. Once released, they enter into fluid sacs which provide cushion between tendons and bones and provoke an inflammatory response. Being the oldest and most common form of arthritis, gout form accumulation of uric acid crystals in joints and nodules in cold parts of the body called tophi.

Once known as a disease of kings, it is now affecting people from every socioeconomic class. It is divided into phases of painful episodes and inter-critical period with no symptom at all. If not properly treated at the right time, the condition may progresses into chronic tophaceous gout. Usually the initial symptom of gout attack appears in the ball of the foot i.e. big toe. There is a sudden inflammation in the metatarsophalangeal joint of the big toe. When gout attacks the big toe, this form of gout is called podagra. Besides big toe gout affects the mid-foot, ankle, knee, wrists, finger joints and helix of the ear. The affected area shows redness and appears shiny due to inflammation of the skin.

Gout attacks usually appear in the morning and reach its maximum peak in six to twenty four hours causing immobility and severe pain. During flare-ups of gout, patient sometimes can't even wear socks. The pain subsides within few days and weeks even if the treatment has not been started yet. It is sometimes characterized by high fever and an increase in the white blood cell count. There are many conditions that decrease solubility of uric acid in blood initiating gout which are infection, trauma to the joint, rapid weight loss, dehydration and acidosis.

Low body temperature also accounts for gout timings and its occurrence in body parts as those body parts are considered cooler. After a painful episode of gout, the inter-critical period starts with no symptoms. Despite an asymptomatic period, uric acid crystals and inflammation still reside in joints.

After the fist attack of gout, a painful episode of gout starts. This painful series of gout proceeds to chronic tophaceous gout, which is characterized by the appearance of nodules due to accumulation of uric acid crystals in colder parts of the body including helix of ear, joints of fingers, toes and elbow.

Formation of tophi affects bone cells (osteoblasts). It affects their growth and causes difficulty in movement. If gout is not managed on time it can halt the quality of life causing dysfunction of joints and immobility. Increase levels of uric acid in the soft tissues and joints not only cause Hyperuricemia but also other serious complications such as chronic inflammation metabolic disorder, cardiovascular disease, kidney dysfunction hypertension and obesity.

2) Who Gets Hyperuricemia And Why?

The primary risk factor for gout is Hyperuricemia and in order to understand gout we must learn the key risk factors that can make anyone susceptible to this painful disease. The incidence of gout increases with age and its prevalence is more common in men than women. Men have higher levels of uric acid in the blood. Fortunately, women have estrogen which is uricosuric in nature and washes out uric acid from the body. So younger women are at lower risk of gout, however, after menopause gout symptoms develop quickly.

Aging also accounts for many medical complications along with susceptibility's to Hyperuricemia and gout. As with aging, functional capacities of the kidney also decrease with time. Vitamin C is also found to have an inverse relationship with uric acid. It is uricosuric in nature but its mechanism is not clear. Research studies reveal the beneficial effect of cherries for gout patients as it is shown to have reduced uric acid levels in gout patients. Now, the lifestyle trends are more advanced and they have increased the risk for gout. These include luxurious habits like alcohol consumption, lack of exercise and diet, which have a strong influence in developing gout.

The most contributing factors which increase the risk of gout are the use of nephrotoxic drugs and diuretics. These medicines cause impaired kidney functions.

Medications such as loop and thiazide diuretics, anti-tuberculosis drugs, cyclosporin and levodopa increase the chances of gout, which is fortunately reversible and the symptoms disappear after discontinuation of therapy.

Low levels of Aspirin inhibit uric acid excretion from the body and high doses reduce the level in the blood. Due to this dual effect of aspirin, it is not recommended in NSAIDs therapy for gout. Diet also affects uric acid level. Consumption of purine rich diet especially red meat and shell fish increases the level of uric acid in the body. Results from various research programs reveals that beef, pork, sea food and lamb in the diet increase the risk of gout by 77% respectively.

However, there is no association of gout with poultry products and protein intake. Plant purines seem to be a safer option in comparison to meat and fish. High alcohol consumption increases levels of uric acid in the blood.

Studies suggest that people who drink beer or spirits everyday are more likely to develop gout than those who drink occasionally. Alcohol interferes with purine metabolism causing a rise in blood uric acid levels. It also lowers body temperature making the body prone to gout attacks. Studies suggest that alcoholics have gout with a very low uric acid level of the blood. Beer has a low alcohol concentration but being rich in purine content increases the chances of Hyperuricemia.

Rich sugar drinks also increase the chances of gout. Fructose is linked to increase uric acid levels in blood. A National health and nutrition examination survey suggest that people who consume more than one sugar drink everyday are more likely to develop gout than those who drink one or two in a month. Also some sweetened fruit juices increase uric acid levels in the blood.

Therefore fructose shares a direct relationship with Hyperuricemia and gout.

In many people there is increased production of uric acid in the body and its levels are high both in urine and the blood. This condition is a genetic defect where a mutation in a gene causes an enzyme defect. This defect increases uric acid overproduction in the body, causing kidney stones and Hyperuricemia.

Patients going through chemotherapy are at increased risk of gout as the killing of tumor cells cause purine breakdown and can initiate gout or stone formation. However, this enzymatic defect is very rare. Studies report symptoms of genetic predisposition in men however its genetic origin is not clearly understood.

High levels of uric acid levels are inherited. SLC2A9, the gene responsible for urate transport regulation, is found to have links with Hyperuricemia. This gene is primarily responsible for the reabsorption of uric acid from the kidney. Mutation of this important gene leads to decreased excretion of uric acid from the body.

The transporter genes for glucose and fructose (GLUT9) also have shown a strong relation to uric acid transport in proximal tubules of the kidney. Genetic polymorphism associated with these genes also influences the levels of uric acid in the blood. Other genes are also reported to have an association with gout, including ABCG2 and SLC17A3.

There is another important factor that affects blood uric acid levels, which is the use of medicines. There are many medicines which increase the levels of uric acid in the blood while there are those which reduce its life. Diuretics are known to increase serum uric acid levels, whereas uricosuric agents and vitamin c reduces the levels in the body.

These medicines interfere with urate transport genes in the proximal tubule of the kidney. Use of thiazide and loop diuretic increases the risk of secondary gout. Patients with organ transplants are at risk of developing gout. Cyclosporin is a risk factor in developing gout with patients of organ transplant. Studies have shown its interaction with transport genes.

Transplant patients develop tophi in many joints thereby making the treatment process complex and painful.

To make the long story short, the prevalence of gout has now increased due to changes in dietary habits, lifestyles, and use of certain medications in daily life. Gout is not fatal but it surely affects the quality of life. The prime objective of therapy is to maintain the quality of life and reduction in uric acid levels. By making some changes in lifestyle and diet, one can make themselves less prone to this painful disease.

With a clear understanding of its mechanism, associated factors which increase its incidence and other health threats associated with high levels of uric acid we can make strategies to control it. Patient education is an important tool in getting the desired outcomes for therapy.

3) The Role Of Hyperuricemia In Other Conditions

The main culprit for gout is Hyperuricemia, but there are many medical conditions in which there are high levels of uric acid. Urolithiasis, a disease in which stones are formed in the kidney or bladder, also occur due to Hyperuricemia and gout. In these conditions, the formation of calcium oxalate crystals along with uric acid crystals takes place.

Several studies suggest that patients with gout are at increased risk of developing calcium oxalate crystals in comparison to patients without symptoms of gout. There are possible chances of kidney damage as a deposition of uric acid crystals in the kidney occur. In kidney damage, uric acid crystals are developing in the proximal tubules and tophi appears on the joints.

The uric acid crystals are not only depositing in proximal tubules of the kidney, but also in other parts of the kidney, initiating an inflammatory response. Studies report the progression of kidney damage with increased levels of uric acid in the blood. Almost

40% of gout patients suffer from renal failure and it accounts for death in 25% of these patients. Patients with gout have more chances of developing kidney and bladder stones.

Kidney complications arise not only due to uric acid crystals but also the presence of calcium oxalate crystals. Increased excretion of uric acid from the body facilitates stone formation in the kidney and bladder. Persistent acidic urine increases the risk of urate deposition thereby favoring gout. Urine uric acid level and creatinine ratios are indicative markers of increased uric acid levels in the body. Such increased levels of uric acid in the body account for metabolic disorders. Studies among different socioeconomic groups suggest an increased risk of metabolic syndrome with increased levels of uric acid in blood.

Hyperuricemia increases the risk of type 2 diabetes in patients, as reported by multiple risk factor trial(MRFIT). Normally, males are more susceptible to develop type 2 diabetes. Not only this, but Hyperuricemia also increases the chances of obesity, and hypertension.

A prevalence study reports the presence of metabolic syndrome in 63% population suffering from gout. High levels of uric acid in the body can attribute to cardiovascular problems. It makes life more complicated in heart patients. Hyperuricemia increases the risk of coronary diseases, heart failure and stroke in patients with gout. High blood pressure patients also suffer from gout.

Studies show that treatments that lower serum uric acid levels also reduce blood pressure during treatment. But unfortunately, high levels of uric acid increase the chances of cardiovascular events because of xanthase oxidase. The overall oxidative stress increases in the body. This enzyme synthesizes uric acid in the body and makes it form free radicals and toxins. It is very common now and recognized as the main and a key factor for gout. Studies suggest the prevalence has increased by 15-20%.

However, studies show that many individuals with asymptomatic Hyperuricemia even develop arthritis. Gout badly affects quality of life in all aspects. There are many complications and medical comorbidities that are associated with gout, making life less functional. Therefore patient education and advice on lifestyle changes could be a great support system in eliminating symptoms and improving quality of life.

Chapter 7: Treating Gout

1) Treating Acute Attacks

Gout can be a life threatening and painful disease if not treated right on time, as discussed in previous chapters. If it is misdiagnosed and treatment is not initiated then it halts the quality of life. It is characterized by inflammation of the joints, tophi and painful gout episodes. In this chapter, we will explore the possible treatment regime and medicines to avoid such painful conditions. However there is still debate on the best regime suitable for the patient.

This chapter contains the best treatment methods and alternatives. In order to get maximum advantage of the content, the patient must discuss this book with an expert physician to alter any medicine or ongoing treatment. An expert physician can suggest the best possible medicine and treatment plan for the patient. Correct diagnosis is very important for the treatment once gout is diagnosed. Painful episodes of pain and immobility can be prevented by taking essential measures.

The treatment of gout is divided into three parts.
1- Treatment of acute gout attacks.
2- Managing Hyperuricemia.
3- Prophylaxis (attack prevention).

Let us discuss them in detail to get an overview on the best treatment regimens available today.

Treatment of acute gout attacks.

The inflammatory response which mediates the crystal induction in the tissues and joints must be stopped right on time to stop the progress of the disease. The important step in the treatment of gout is to stop the inflammation before it creates complications. Usually treatment is started just after the first sign appears. If the treatment is delayed or not started because of any misdiagnosis then it is a lifelong treatment which needs proper care and attention. If the disease has progressed, taking medicines won't ease the pain. If the patient waits for few hours and then takes the medicine he or she might get relief after a few days, in contrast to those patients who react just after the first attack and get instant relief within hours. So patients must be well educated and well informed about the disease and must keep medicines with them all the time. It is advised to keep some medicines in the workplace, car, near the bed side, purse or anywhere as a first aid.

Medicines Used to treat Acute Gout Attack

a) Non-Steroidal Anti Inflammatory Drugs (NSAIDs)

The first line of agent used in the treatment of acute gout attacks is non-steroidal anti-inflammatory drugs or NSAIDs. The key point in treating gout attacks is to halt the inflammatory process before it progresses, and here comes the NSAIDs to the rescue. This group of medicines suppresses inflammation and reduces swelling. The mechanism of action of NSAIDs is quite simple; they block cyclooxygenase (COX) enzyme which triggers inflammation in the cells. There are two classes of NSAIDs primarily called selective NSAIDs and non-selective NSAIDs. Non-selective class of NSAIDs are used for the treatment of gout. Three different COX enzymes are working in the human body and non-selective NSAIDs blocks COX-1 and COX-2 enzymes in the body. COX-2 inhibitors, or selective NSAIDs, are another class of NSAIDs used to treat gout. These medicines block COX-2 enzyme and inhibit the inflammatory process. Apparently, selective NSAIDs have gained popularity over non-selective NSAIDs, as they have fewer side effects and are mild on the gastric tract. But non-selective NSAIDs are still used to treat gout regardless of their harmful effect on the gastrointestinal tract.

NSAIDs Used to Treat Acute Gout Attacks

The most commonly prescribed NSAIDs approved by the U.S Food and Drug Administration are:

Indomethacin
Available by the trade names of:
Apo- Indomethacin ®, Indameth ®, Indocin ®,Indacid ® and Novo-Methacin ®.

Naproxen
Available by the trade names of:
Aleve®, Naprosyn®,Anaprox®, Anaprox DS ®,Novo-Naprox ®, and Naprelan ®.

Sulindac
Available by the trade names of:
Clinoril ®, Aclin ®,Apo-Sulin ® and Novo-Sundac ®.

One of the selective NSAIDs used for the treatment of gout is celecoxib. It is very gentle on the gastrointestinal tract. It is gaining popularity for the treatment of gout but not yet approved by FDA for this use. Some of the effective NSAIDs are as under:

Celecoxib
Available by the trade names of:
Celebrex ® and Celebra ®

Ibuprofen
Available by the trade names of:
Motrin ®, Advil ®, Ibu-Tab200 ®, Tab-Profen ®, Profen ®, ACT-3 ®, Brufen ®, IBU ®,
Ibu-Tabs ® and Novo-Profen ®.

Ketoprofen
Available by the trade names of:
Orudis ®,Actron ®,Apo-Keto ®,Novo-Keto ® and Rhodis ®

Piroxicam
Available by the trade names of:
Feldene ®,Apo-Piroxicam ® and Novo-Piroxicam ®

Diclofenac
 Available by the trade names of:
 Cataflam ®, Voltaren ® and Solaraze ®.

Ibuprofen, Naproxen and Ketoprofen are over the counter medicines available without prescription in the U.S and many countries of the world. So in that case, if someone has a sudden onset of pain these medicines are a good choice and easily available if prescription medicines are not available at that time.

But it should be discussed along with other precautions with the physician as not all the medicines suit everyone. Besides the appropriate use, its dose should also be discussed with the physician. The dose used to treat gout is high as compared to the dose printed on the label of the strip. Immediate release formula of medicine is recommended as compared to sustained release. In case of any confusion, a pharmacist must be consulted.

Taking NSAIDs

Doses prescribed for gout attacks are as follows, however patients should always follow the advice of a doctor.

Indomethacin
The initial dose of Indomethacin is 100mg after the first symptoms of gout followed by 50 mg three times a day. The dose must not be exceeded more than 200mg per day. Stop taking medicine when the pain subsides.

Naproxen

The starting dose is 750mg after the first sign of symptoms followed by 250mg every eight hours. The dose must be reduced after two or three days as the symptoms subside. Don't take more than 750mg after the first day and not more than 10 days.

Sulindac

Initial dose is 200mg twice a day. The dose must be reduced after two or three days after the symptoms subside. Dose must exceed more than 400mg and not more than seven days.

Warning about NSAIDs

NSAIDs should be used with caution, especially over the counter medicines. So it is important to discuss them with your physician before taking them or changing them. Patient education about these medicines is very important and one must read FDA guidelines about these medicines written in the Appendix B. Patients need to be educated about the medicinal use; its dose; taking time and patients must make the habit of reading labels and prescribing information for better understanding. It's important to get counseling from a physician or pharmacist in case of any confusion. NSAIDs are known to cause gastrointestinal irritations, bleeding, ulcers and perforations.

The situation gets worst in case of poor health, alcohol consumption, aspirin, aspirin-containing products, corticosteroids and anti-coagulants. The risk of gastric bleeding is high and can happen with or without any symptoms, which could be fatal. Heart attack or stroke is another life threatening side effect of NSAIDs. People taking these medicines for a long period of time are more at risk of heart attack and stroke, whereas people who are heart patients are at greater risk. It is recommended not to use any NSAIDs before or after any heart surgery.

These life threatening side effects makes NSAIDs inappropriate for long-term treatment. The best way to deal with this issue is to take NSAIDs right after the first symptom, which will reduce its treatment time.

NSAIDs are contraindicated or inhibited in the following conditions:
1 – Elderly,
2 - Renal impairment,
3 - liver problem,
4 - Heart problem,
5 - Peptic ulcer,
6 - Stomach/Heartburn problems,
7 - Pregnancy,
8 - Bleeding problems,
9 - Diuretics therapy,
10 - Anticoagulant therapy.

Uric acid lowering medicine Probenecid, decreases NSAIDs excretion from the body, thus making them extremely harmful. It also causes gastric bleeding. A patient taking Probenecid must consult with their physicians before taking NSAIDs. The dose must be adjusted to avoid any possible adverse drug interaction. NSAIDs also cause allergic reactions in some people, such as facial swelling or difficulty in breathing. Immediately stop taking these medicines and call a physician for first aid.

b) Colchicine

Colchicines are the most commonly prescribed medicine for the treatment of acute gout. Before NSAIDs were discovered, Colchicine was the only drug of choice in acute gout. Colchicine is isolated from the bulb of the autumn crocus flower and does not inhibit COX enzymes, although it disrupts the movement of white blood cells. By doing so, they are unable to enter the cell and attack uric acid crystals. It helps protect white blood cells that are killed during the therapy to reduce inflammation. However, Colchicine is less effective in the treatment of gout compared to NSAIDs. Its elimination is very slow from the body therefore there are more chances of its buildup in the body causing harmful effects. It's extremely harmful when taken in high doses.

Nausea, vomiting, diarrhea are common side effects of Colchicine. In the past, Colchicine was used in high doses to treat acute gout. But now it's given in low doses as they are as effective as high doses but with side effects. However, it's used in case the patient can't tolerate NSAIDs. Despite all these facts, Colchicine is a good choice in case there is confusion in the diagnosis of gout. Colchicine is an emergency drug, which can be used in prophylaxis. Its high and low doses are described as follows, although dose must be adjusted and patients need to consult with a physician before taking them.

Low Dose Method
Low dose of Colchicine is.5mg or .6mg three or four times a day. The dose must not exceed more than 6mg. Discontinue medicine when the pain subsides.

High Dose Method (not recommended)
0.6mg tablet after the first attack followed by every hour till the pain subsides. The dose must not exceed more than 6mg.

Warnings about Colchicine:
One must wait for three days after taking a high dose of Colchicine. As Colchicine eliminates slowly from the body to avoid build up one must wait for the levels to fall. More than 6mg cause a fatal condition and must be avoided. If Colchicine is used for prophylaxis then it must not be given for acute treatment, as there are risks of overdose. It is eliminated by the kidney and liver. People with kidney and liver problems are at more risk of developing toxic levels of Colchicine in the body. Patients with kidney or liver disease must consult their physician before taking Colchicine. Colchicine can suppress bone marrow, therefore it can't be prescribed in this condition. It can be given by injection but this method is banned in U.S.

c) Other Medication for Acute Gout Attack

If the patient can't tolerate the above mentioned medicines then second and third line agents are used. These medicines have more side effects and are much more expensive. Some of these alternatives are discussed below.

Corticosteroids
Being the most potent anti-inflammatory agents they work by suppressing the immune system. When injected they provide fast relief from pain as compared to any treatment options available.

They are the best drug of choice in many cases such as NSAIDs and Colchicine intolerance, severe attacks, multi joint attacks or when gout is left untreated. They can be directly introduced into the joint, which makes them very effective. But this technique is very painful and needs an expert handling. It's very difficult to administer in hand and foot joints and there is also risk of crystallization of the medicine itself which can make the situation worse. That's why they are given intra muscularly (in muscle) or intravenously (in vein) which is equally effective. Orally they are less effective and act very slowly.

d) ACTH (Adrenocorticotropic hormone or corticotrophins)

Our pituitary gland secretes this hormone, which is found to be very effective in treating gout. It's marketed by the trade name of Crtrosyn® which is its synthetic version. Researchers suggest that this hormone is effective more than Indomethacin. It is very expensive and can only be given via injection. It is a fortunate solution for people with congestive heart failure, chronic kidney failures and those who are not responding to any above mentioned treatment regimes.

e) Painkillers

Among the group of painkillers, narcotics are used for the treatment of acute gout. But unfortunately they can't reduce pain and inflammation and are highly addictive.

f) Rest

Rest is very important for gout patients as moving and stressing the joint can initiate the pain due to the presence of uric acid crystals in the joint and soft tissues. It increases inflammation and reduces the quality of life. Rest for one to two days will ease the pain and applying ice on the affected joint would also help.

2) Managing Hyperuricemia

First we discussed how to treat gout attack but as it is said prevention is better than cure so now we will discuss how to prevent gout attacks. As we know, gout occurs due to accumulation of uric acid crystals in the joint and soft tissues due to high levels of uric acid in the body. So apparently, reducing the levels of uric acid might help. But unfortunately, it is a lifelong therapy with lots of precautions throughout their life. The fact that it is baseless to treat asymptomatic Hyperuricemia is now challenged. There are also questions about when to treat Hyperuricemia and gout.

Data collected from research suggests that treatment must be started right after the first attack. Also, family history plays an important role. If you have high levels of uric acid in the blood there is the likelihood of developing gout. Treatment must start after tophi formation to prevent further damage. Similarly, uric acid levels in the blood must be checked after the attack. If uric acid levels are higher than 12mg/dl for men or 10mg/dl for women, treatment must be started as soon as possible.

There are two classes of drugs used in the management of gout. These medications as described as follows.

Xanthine Oxidase Inhibitor Drugs

These drugs interfere with the metabolic processes, which create uric acid as an end product. They inhibit the enzyme Xanthine Oxidase. Allopurinol is a Xanthine Oxidase inhibitor and a drug of choice in the management of painful episodes of gout. It is given once daily and has less side effects. It works in both conditions of Hyperuricemia, that have over production and underexcretion. 20% of patients might have side effects, which could be serious and life threatening. These side effects include rash, fever, pale skin and eyes. In case of any of these symptoms consult the physician immediately. Possible drug interactions reported are with an immunosuppressant drug azathioprine.

It is used for patients with organ transplant and inflammatory bowel disease. Allopurinol also interacts with mercaptopurine, which is used in leukemia patients. Allopurinol is not recommended in these patients taking mercaptopurine. The Xanthine Oxidase inhibitor class has three more drugs but they are in clinical trial phase.

Febuxostat among the three is found to be more promising and beneficial. Its marketed in Europe by the trade name of Adenuric®, but it is in clinical trials in the U.S. This drug is considered a replacement of Allopurinol, since it has fewer side effects.

Uricosuric Drugs

This class of drug helps the body to filter and excrete uric acid with the help of a kidney. These drugs are considered as a great substitute for Allopurinol. However, there is a great risk of kidney stones in patients taking uricosuric drugs.

During the therapy, the concentration of uric acid is higher in the kidney and, urinary tract can result in kidney stone formation. It could be prevented by drinking two or three liters of water every day. A 24 hour urine test is recommended after starting uricosuric drugs. Make sure urine is not acidic, as acidic urine indicates uric acid crystals. Ask your doctor and drink as much water as possible to wash out the toxin from the body.

Uricosuric drugs interfere with antibiotics, which might be dangerous. They also alter the potency of NSAIDs and increase their concentration causing toxic side effects. Probenecid, Sulfinpyrazone and Benzbromarone are uricosuric agents used for the treatment. However, Sulfinpyrazone is not available in the U.S. Other medications, namely Micronised fenofibrate, losartan and amlodipine are also effective uricosuric drugs.

Uric Acid Lowering Drug Dosages

Allopurinol
Marketed by the trade name of Lopurin®, Apo-Allopurinol®,Zyloprim®, and Allorin®. Starting dose is 100mg/day for a week then followed by 200mg/day for the second week and 300mg/day for the third week. The dose must not be exceeded more than 800mg/day.

Febuxostat
Marketed by trade name of Adenuric® starting dose is 80mg once daily. Then if the serum uric acid levels are more than 6mg/dl then 120mg once daily. The dose must not exceed 120mg/day.

Probenecid
Probenecid is marketed by the trade names of Benemid®,Probalan®, and Benuryl®. Its starting dose is given 250mg/day, which is increased by two to three weeks for 1000mg/day. 500mg tablet is given twice a day but the dose is increased gradually to prevent kidney stones. Maximum dose is 3000mg/day and must not exceed this limit.

Sulfinpyrazone
Sulfinpyrazone is marketed by the trade names of Anturane®,and

Anturan®. Initial dose is given 100mg once a day which is later on increased to twice a day after two or three weeks. The dose is gradually increased to three times a day after three weeks. The purpose behind this slow dose increase is to prevent kidney stones. Don't exceed the dose more than 400mg/day.

Benzbromarone
Benzbromarone is withdrawn from the market because of its fatal liver failure adverse effect. However, it's a powerful uricosuric agent despite of its life threatening adverse effect. It also works in people with kidney failure, however the patient needs to be monitored in case of taking this medicine.

Uric Acid Lowering Medications

Medicines used to lower uric acid in the body decrease the risk of gout attacks. However, variations in uric acid levels increase the risk of gout.

Do's And Don'ts Of Uric Acid Therapy

1-During or after a gout attack don't take these medicines, as during these attacks levels of uric acid fluctuates which can increase uric acid levels in the body, increasing risk of another attack. So in that case wait for two or three weeks till uric acid levels calm down. If an attack occurs during the treatment, don't stop taking medication. If the medication is discontinued or dose is changed then this might fluctuate uric acid levels leading to painful episodes of gout.

2- Always start these medicines with minimum dose and then gradually increase over weeks to avoid any risk of kidney stones.

3- Uricosuric agents might not stop the attacks at once but sometimes they increase their frequency. So patient must not be discouraged and need to stick to it. Treatment is long and might go for six months or a year to lower the levels. It must be remembered, that high uric acid levels will not only be present in the blood but everywhere in the body so it will take time to flush out the toxin and stabilizes its concentration in the body.

The most important among these factors is poor patient compliance in case they don't get desired results within a short period; they think the medicines are not working and discontinue them. So patient education is very important they must stick to the regime to improve the quality of life.

Follow Up

Follow up is very important in treatment regarding uric acid lowering medications. The Serum uric acid level must be checked every two or four weeks after three to six months of therapy. The dose must be adjusted according to the levels to get the desired level in the body.

The same way diabetic patients get their blood sugar levels checked, gout patients must also know their serum uric acid levels. Patient education plays an important role in improving their wellbeing and quality of life. Usually, serum uric acid levels below 6mg/dl (360μmol/lit) are considered a target level of uric acid lowering treatment.

However, 5mg/dl (278μmol/lit) is suggested by British Society for Rheumatology guidelines. Research reveals that a reduction in uric acid level up to 4mg/dl (222μmol/lit) reduces the tophi size incredibly. Levels lower than 2.16mg/dl (120μmol/lit) can trigger other health problems in the body. As soon as the desired target levels are achieved, physicians recommend annual testing and dose adjustments.

As we know, uric acid level keep fluctuating so timely testing is required to keep the target levels in the body. However, there is no best testing time given anywhere in the guidelines. Physicians also recommend combination therapy including Xanthine Oxidase inhibitor drugs and uricosuric drugs for patients with high levels of uric acid in the body. It's also proving to be effective for patients who don't respond to single drug therapy for lowering uric acid levels in the body.

Thus, this combination therapy works in both conditions of overproduction and under excretion of uric acid. The patient must be educated to read the labels and prescription information before taking any medicine and must consult the physician or pharmacist in case of any confusion.

3) Prophylaxis - Attack Prevention

In this part we will learn to take preventive measures against high levels of uric acid in the blood. Uricosuric agents dissolve uric acid in the blood and get them eliminated from the kidney. This process increases the levels and frequency of painful attacks.

For that purpose, prophylaxis are used for prevention of such painful episodes. In prophylaxis treatment regime a low dose is given to the patient to prevent further attacks. In the case of uricosuric agents, therapy prophylactic treatment is recommended. Colchicine is the drug of choice in prophylaxis. Since it causes side effects at high doses, its low dose causes less side effects making it suitable for therapy.

As compared to NSAIDs it's a much safer approach in long-term treatment. In case the patient is not tolerant to Colchicine, then low doses of NSAIDs are given. This is a temporary treatment and it works with uricosuric agents in lowering the uric acid levels in the body. Its main purpose is to minimize the frequency of attacks. There are contradictions of the treatment time period, as three months or a year are given according to some experts. However, prophylaxis must be continued till the normal serum uric acid level target is achieved which is less than 6mg/dl or 360μmol/lit.

After the tophi disappears and the patient doesn't have a gout attack for approximately six months, then it is discontinued. The time period of prophylaxis is dependable on the previous attacks and their frequency. As more attacks suggest long-term prophylaxis, treatment is required. If after three months attack symptoms appear, then go on treatment for another three months till the symptoms subside.

One must keep in mind that self-medication is as harmful as poisoning oneself. Many drugs interfere with each other and one must consult an expert physician before taking any medicine or dosage change.

Prophylaxis Dosing:

Colchicine: 0.5mg-1.8mg a day

Indomethacin: 25mg twice a day for six months

Naproxen: 250mg once daily

N.B Someone taking Colchicine for a prophylaxis treatment must not take it for acute attacks, as it increases the risk of over-dosing. In case of any confusion consult the physician immediately.

Alternative Treatments

An expert with an experience of more than 45 years has formulated his own method of treating gout. According to the experts, gout attack is reversed quickly when treated with a combination of drugs at the same time. According to experts, one must start uricosuric agent therapy right after the first attack. Waiting is baseless and start the therapy with a very low dose and then increase the dose gradually to get the desired target levels of uric acid in the body.

Treatment Regime

1- Low dose Colchicine: Patient is advised to take .6mg of Colchicine four times a day till the dosage of 6mg is achieved and pain subsides completely.

2- Taking an NSAID at the same time: Take an NSAID along with it according to medical history and health condition.

3- Use of Intra-Muscular Injection of Corticosteroid: A Corticosteroid such as methyl prednisolone (available by the trade name of DepoMedrol®) is used. They are strong anti-inflammatory agents and are very effective when given by injection (parenteral route of administration).

4- Painkillers: Painkillers such as dextropropoxyphene (available by trade names of Darvocet-N®. Balacet®. Di-gesic®) and acetaminophen or paracetamol (Tylenol®) with codeine can also be given.

5- In case of not taking a Uricosuric drug: If this is the case then start taking the medicine at a low dose. Don't wait for three weeks, start a small dose and gradually increase it to maintain desired target levels.

According to experts, if uricosuric therapy is started then it's baseless to go for prophylaxis. This also means that one should not leave asymptomatic hyperuricemia untreated, as this is just waiting for it to develop into a more severe form.

4) Gout Management At a Glance

Acute attacks are prevented by taking an NSAIDs or Colchicine, as suggested by the physician. The most important preventive measure is to take medicine right after the first attack and don't neglect the symptoms. As a first aid keep some of the medicines handy at your work place, car and bed side to prevent a sudden attack. Consult with your physician about the medicines and their dosage in case of sudden attack.

With this habit you will learn to stop the attack in an hour or so without building tension and immobility and can improve your own wellbeing. In case of managing Hyperuricemia, Uricosuric drug therapy is started two to three weeks after the last attack. The key is to stick to this regime. It's started with a low dose, which is gradually increased to avoid any further health complications like kidney stones. If an attack occurs during the treatment don't stop or change the dosage and stick to the already set regime. One must keep in mind that uricosuric agents may take several months to a year to decrease uric acid levels in the body so the main key point is to stick with the therapy no matter what. Along with a uricosuric agent therapy it is advised to start a prophylactic treatment. Colchicine, Indomethacin or Naproxen are given at low doses.

The therapy might last for three to six months or may be a year depending on frequency of previous attacks.

1- Stopping a Gout Attack: Initiate treatment right after the first attack. The prime purpose is to reduce inflammation the root cause of gout. Delayed treatment might result in another painful episode of gout.
Medications:
Most commonly used NSAIDs: Indomethacin, Naproxen or Sulindac.
Cox-2 inhibitors: Celecoxib

2- Management of Hyperuricemia: Higher levels of uric acid in the body develop gout. Therefore the medicines used in this phase work by lowering uric acid levels in the body to normal levels i.e. 6mg/dl (360μmol/lit)
Medications:

Uric Acid lowering Medications: Allopurinol and Febuxostat
Drugs to lower Uric acid excretion: Probenecid and
Sulfinpyrazone

Directions for Medications:

1- Before starting a treatment, a wait of two or three weeks is
recommended.
2- Therapy starts with a low dose followed by gradual increase in
the dose.
3- In case of any side effects, consult the physician immediately.
4- During an attack, don't discontinue the medications.
5- Prophylaxis must be used to prevent any chances of future
attack.
6- Uric acid levels must be checked frequently during treatment
and after getting the desired target levels, annual checkups are
mandatory.

Prophylaxis: Here it must be kept in mind that during the
prophylaxis, gout attacks might increase in frequency. In that
case, the patient must be encouraged to take the medication with
the correct dosage and stick to this treatment regime. The first
treatment is done for three months but if any attack occurs in
between, treatment might prolong for a year to get the desires
results.

Medication:
Colchicine: In low doses
NSAIDs: Ibuprofen, Ketoprofen, Piroxicam or Diclofenac.
Alternative medications: Colchicine, Corticosteroids or ACTH.

Medicines must be discussed with a physician and dose must be
adjusted. In case of any allergic reaction or sign of side effects,
consult physician. The physician must educate the patient about
the dosage, warnings and possible side effects associated with the
medication. The medication must not be used more than its
required safety dose.

Direction about Probenecid and Sulfinpyrazone:

1- In order to minimize the risk of kidney stones, a 24 hour urine analysis is required before treatment.
2- Those patients with already higher levels or overproduction of uric acid should not be prescribed these medications.
3- Drink maximum water, at least 2-3 liters per day, to wash out toxins and for a healthy kidney.
4- Urine pH must be checked regularly. In case of an acidic urine or pH under 6 consult with the physician.

Alternate options: Naproxen or Indomethacin in a low dose.

Medications must be taken according to the prescribing information and as suggested by the physician. Discuss the medicines that should be taken in case of an emergency in acute gout attack with the correct dose. The patient must be educated to read the labels properly and all the warnings on the label. Self-medication must be avoided as it could be fatal and life threatening in many cases.

Keep all the medications handy in the car, in the office and near the bed to deal with an emergency pain of an acute attack. In case of attack don't stop the medicine and continue taking it. As the amount of uric acid builds up, not only in the blood but in the whole body, it will take a lot of time to excrete out from the body. The patient must be encouraged to not lose hope in that case and stick to the treatment regime and religiously follow it for a healthy life.

Chapter 8: Surgical Treatments

This chapter is targeted to cover large piece of information related to surgical treatments. What is surgery? Its types, its targeted points and results, with advantages and disadvantages associated with it. The reason to add such detailed information related to surgery is that several disorders require surgeries. Particularly, arthritis and gouty arthritis patients have to undergo surgeries at critical situations.

A detailed overview of surgeries, their types, possible organs of surgeries and other points should be handy for readers. Additionally, the readers will be benefited with this book more intensely.

1) Surgery

It is a medical field that deals with operative and instrumental techniques to treat, explore, identify and the diagnosis of disease, its course, underlying pathology and extent. Sometimes it also helps in determining the prognosis of a disease.

2) Types of surgery

Surgery is divided further according to its techniques and the organ involved.

According To Techniques And Method they are classified as follows:

(i) Open surgery involving laparotomy (a large incision is made on the abdomen to reach the underlying organs, used for both diagnosis and treatment of diseases).

(ii) Minimal invasive surgeries such as laparoscopic surgery. This surgery is performed with the help of video assisted camera and ports (small plastic tubes). Small incisions are made and the ports and the camera are inserted through these incisions inside the abdomen to visualize the abdominal organs.

(iii) Microscopic surgeries: it involves the combination of minimal invasive surgery and highly sensitive and advanced microscopes to visualize the most sensitive tissues or organs with accuracy e.g. spinal surgeries.

(iv) Elective surgery: based on patient request such as cosmetic surgeries (mostly done to improve the appearance of the structure (face surgeries, nose surgery to improve appearance looks) or to improve the functioning (example nose surgery to remove any bone defect such as deviated nasal septum) or removing deformities e.g. cleft lip. cleft palate.

(v) Emergency surgery: is performed to save the life of a patient, organ or limb (body part) it mostly includes gastrointestinal surgeries to relieve intestinal obstruction, removal of appendix etc.

3) Surgery -Why And Why Not?

Advantages of surgery

(1) Fast method for dealing with pathological condition of organs

(2) Helps the diagnosis through exploratory surgery

(3) Where medical treatment is no longer helpful, surgery is used to explore further options of treatment using invasive and noninvasive techniques

(4) It also helps in improving the life and appearance of different body parts
(5) Laparoscopic surgery reduced the hemorrhage, less pain less use of medications, less hospital stay and patient can return to daily life activities soon. A small incision leads to minimal or no scaring.

Disadvantages of surgery

(1) Hemorrhage (blood loss): Primary hemorrhage: can occur immediately at the time of surgery,
Reactionary hemorrhage: within 24 hours of surgery,
Secondary hemorrhage: several days after surgery,

(2) Wound complications such as:
Infection: incidence of infection depends upon the type of surgery and the risk of infection (poor nutrition, diabetes, anemia, uremia and reduced immunity increases the risk of infection),

(3) Hematoma (collection of blood and clot): imperfect hemostasis (normal body metabolism) causes collection of blood and clots in the wound which increases the risk of wound infection,

(4) Seroma (localized collection of serous fluid): seromas mostly form where skin flaps have been raised e.g. groin and axilla where lymphatics have been divided,

(5) Wound dehiscence: It is partial or total disruption of any or all layers of the operative wound, factors that cause wound dehiscence are: LOCAL: inadequate closure of wound, raised intra-abdominal pressure and improper wound healing.

SYSTEMIC: age above 60 years, diabetes mellitus, sepsis, immune suppression and malnutrition,

(6) Pus formation,

(7) Pain,

(8) Cardiovascular compromise such as heart failure (inability of the heart to pump enough blood to meet the requirement of the body), DVT (deep venous thrombosis) thrombosis of deep veins of legs occurs due to venous stasis, hyper coagulability and vessel wall injury, myocardial infarction (necrosis/death of heart muscles), arrhythmias (increase heart rate), angina (pain in chest due to heart diseases) etc.,

(9) Respiratory complications: most common cause of death in patients above 60 years,

(10) Atelectasis (collapse of lung): it mostly occurs in first 48 hours. Anesthesia may increase bronchial secretions and decrease ciliary action, there by retaining the mucous in the bronchi, blocking the smaller bronchi and resulting in the absorption of alveolar air, which results in the collapse of an area of the lung followed by infection. Minoratelectasis manifests as pyrexia, dyspnea, tachycardia and fever. Severe form accompanied by cyanosis and respiratory collapse,

(11) Pulmonary aspiration: aspiration may occur during induction or termination of anesthesia,

(12) Pneumonia: post-operative pneumonia is a common complication after surgery, host defense is very weak after surgery and the patient may not be able to cough effectively to clear the bronchial tree and bacteria can also reach the lungs by inhalation from the respirator which leads to fever, tachypnea, increased secretions and consolidation of lungs,

(13) Pulmonary embolism,

(14) Pulmonary edema,

(15) Pulmonary effusion & Pneumothorax: formation of a small amount of pleural effusion is very common after abdominal procedures which suggests sub diaphragmatic inflammation,

(16) GIT complications (bowl obstruction, hepatic dysfunction, constipation, fecal impaction, postoperative ileuses),

(17) Urinary tract infection: infection can easily enter urinary tract through the catheter,

(18) Acute renal shut down (failure of kidneys to perform its function leading to build up of harmful substance in the body),

(19) Urinary retention: a very common surgical complication a palpable bladder is present in examination,

(20) Complications of surgical drains: large rigid drains erode in to adjacent viscera causing fistula formation and bleeding, increase the rate of infection and promote leakage,

(21) CNS complications: stroke, confusion, fits,

(22) Fever: presence of post-operative fever indicates either one of following:

- Wound: discharge, pus or infection in the wound can be the cause of fever.

- Chest infections: chest infections mostly occur after surgery leading to pyrexia (fever)

- Urinary tract infection (UTI): UTI may occur between 5-7 days after surgery, they also cause fever.

Complications relating to different surgeries are increased if the patient has pre-existing diseases, such as COPD, asthma, pulmonary fibrosis etc.

4) Negative Aspects of Surgical Removal of Gout

Gout is the intra articular deposition of urate crystals due to disorder of urate metabolism, mostly affecting first MTP joint (podagra) present with sudden excruciating joint pain along with erythematous, swollen and tender joint. Usually medical treatment is the first line treatment including NSAIDS (e.g., Indomethacin), Colchicine, and steroids when NSAIDS are not effective or contraindicated. Allopurinol and probenecid are used for disorders in urate metabolism for over producers and under secretors vice versa.

If medical treatment is not effective, only then surgery is performed but it has its own complications such as:

- Infection: common complication of surgery while removing tophi sometimes joint become infected

- Joint fusion: surgical complications sometimes lead to joint fusion joint become stiff tender.

- Pain and disability, pain and loss of functioning of joint is a very common complication.

Chapter 9: Lifestyle Changes Required for Gout

Special Note

The purpose of this chapter is to guide you to make some positive changes in your life, which will be worth it in the end. The sole purpose lies in encouraging you to be healthy and enjoy life with full enthusiasm. Gout treatments are usually life-long and it's very important to not lose hope and stick to the regime with a healthy lifestyle. Formerly known as the disease that only affected the wealthy classes, it now affects almost everyone.

As we have learned already, the main culprit is uric acid which is formed as a waste product of purine metabolism, which causes these high levels resulting in Hyperuricemia and gout. This important chemical is supposed to be an antioxidant as well and lowering its levels also gives rise to serious health threats. However, our generation is fortunate enough to control this emerging phenomenon which is on the rise these days. As a lot of research has been done on how to control this painful monster snatching all the energy from the body, it has been revealed that there are certain measures which can help to control gout.

There is no magic potion to correct it overnight but it's you, your will power and your working and coordination with physicians and taking positive health measures and changes in your lifestyle that can make a change.

Emotional Help
We have discussed in earlier chapters that gout treatment is lifelong and takes a lot of time. Patience is the only key to survive

in the long run, therefore it's very important to provide moral support to the patient. As gout affects almost all areas of life, sometimes it becomes very difficult to handle such chronic illness without the support of physician and family.

Changes in life are not easy to take, especially when they come with the fear of the future. What will happen when we grow older, what if the medicines don't react well etc. However, with time, people learn to combat this disease with a good counseling, moral support of family and friends and changes in lifestyle.

Here is a reminder of certain lifestyle changes one should make for a healthy well-being.

1) Lifestyle Recommendations to Gout Patients

a) Dietary Recommendations

As we know, DNA breaks down into nucleic acid and forms purine which later breaks down into uric acid. Purine rich diet consumption also gives rise to high uric acid in the body. This in turn increases the load on the kidney to excrete huge amounts of uric acid. This may give rise to further complications and kidney impairment. Purines don't only come from animal cells but also plant cells. Lots of researchers reveal that plant purines are safe in comparison to meat and fish purines. Not all the purine containing foods are harmful and dairy products with purine actually help us to lower our risk of gout. Dietitians recommend lowering daily purine intake to around 150 milligrams.

The purine rich food having 1,000mg per 3.5 ounce serving are brains, gravies, kidney, liver, sardines and sweet breads. Whereas foods with 100mg per 3.5 ounce servings are asparagus, bacon, beef, bluefish, calf tongue, carp, cauliflower, chicken, chicken, soup, codfish, crab, duck, goose, lamb, lentils, mushrooms, mutton, navy beans, peas, pork, rabbit, salmon, sheep, spinach, tuna , turkey and trout. We know that we do need small and healthy amounts of purine in our body to protect our blood vessels and act as an antioxidant.

b) Critical Dietary Inclusions

Low Fat Dairy products
Diet containing low fat actually decreases the risk of gout. Yogurt and skimmed milk are found to be beneficial in lowering the risk.

Fresh Fruits and Vegetables
One must add fresh fruits and vegetables in their diet to reduce the risk of gout. Fruits rich in vitamin C are proving to be beneficial in reducing gout. Vitamin C rich fruits include kiwi, mango, guava and berries.

Vitamins
Those who take vitamins daily are at a lower risk of developing gout. The recommended daily dose of vitamin C is 500-1000mg which reduces the risk of gout and decreases uric acid in the body. Vitamin C is contraindicated in mega doses and proves to be effective in low doses. The dose must not exceed 1500mg per day.

Cherries
Cherries are found to be an important antioxidant in the management of gout. Studies reveal that cherries decrease serum uric acid levels significantly. Cherries also reduce inflammation in the body, therefore proving to be an important gout remedy.

Nuts, Seeds & Legumes
Nuts, seeds and legumes have proven their efficacy not only for gout but also insulin resistance. Nuts, seeds and legumes must be added in diet to improve health.

Stay Hydrated
Water is an elixir of life and many dietitians suggest drinking 2-3 liters of water daily. Increase the intake if you are exercising on a

daily basis. As we all know water is helpful in transporting nutrients and wastes and regulates our body temperature and comforts joints. Lack of water in the body brings a lot of health problems including kidney stones and constipation. Therefore, keep your body hydrated to flush out toxins and keep uric acid levels normal in the body.

c) Some of the dietary exclusions are as follows

Animal Derived Purines
Animal derived protein sources, such as red meat and seafood, are shown to increase the pain. Those with preexisting gout must also take caution and don't eat such foods. However, purine rich vegetables are not much harmful in comparison. Foods such as processed meat, organ meat, red meats, shellfish, yeasts, oily fishes and sardines have high purine content.

Soft Drinks
Soft drinks usually have a high content of sugar and therefore must be avoided to reduce the risk of gout. Some soft drinks also contain a huge amount of artificial sweeteners, which increase the risk.

In order to give an idea of diet a sample of the diet is given below.

Breakfast:
Papaya, rose water, lime and natural yogurt are supposed to be taken for breakfast. As yogurt contains essential protein and antioxidants, being a low fat dairy it is beneficial for health. Papaya is a good source of vitamin C and helps in reducing the risk of gout. Lemon, being a detoxifying and cleansing agent, is also rich in huge amount of vitamin C. They boost overall immunity of the body. You can also take cereals with skimmed milk or whole wheat.

Lunch

Converting to a vegetarian diet can make it easy for most of the patients to prevent gout. As vegetables have low purine levels, they help in reducing uric acid in the body. Salads and roasted vegetables like roast pumpkin and beetroot salad with a mix of green vegetables are recommended. You can eat lean meat, poultry, or fish along with a sandwich or whole wheat bread.

Dinner

A vegetable rich diet cleanses the body and boosts immunity. They have been traditionally used to reduce the risk of gout in many countries. Any vegetable soup would be highly nutritious and healthy. Red lentils will fill the need for protein. 2-3ounces of roasted chicken, steamed vegetables and baked potatoes will be a healthier mix.

Snacks

Patients with gout can eat a low purine salad vegetable based snack. Carrot sticks, chickpeas and avocado could be used. Fruit salads including cherries, kiwi, guava and berries would be very nutritious. It can be accompanied by yogurt and mixed nuts.

Beverages

Make a cherry juice or eat it alone. Cherry being an antioxidant and anti-inflammatory would ease the pain and improve immunity. Celery and ginger juice is also recommended, as ginger being anti-inflammatory reduces inflammation and celery is a diuretic which helps cleanse the body to offload the burden.

2) Exercise and Gout

Exercises are very important when living with gout. A no exercise routine will make the situation worse and increase the pain frequency. It's very painful to move and immobility and lack of movement are a few attributes associated with gout. This lazy routine ends up in weak and fragile muscles and less flexibility. Exercise is crucial for health otherwise the pain will amplify and make things more complicated. The exercise proves to be beneficial in faster healing and recovery from gout. When properly done, exercise improves stamina, energy and helps you keep in good shape. It's also important in maintaining a healthy body weight. Exercise helps in reversing the effects of gout and helps build up strong muscles. After a few weeks, you will notice an increase in stamina and energy. Some of the exercises are described below which will help you lower your uric acid levels as well as getting a sense of wellbeing. It is important to consult with a physician before starting any exercise for best results.

Low Impact Cardio Exercise
Cardio exercises not only improve lung function capacity but also prove to be helpful in utilizing oxygen for removing acids from the body. These exercises also strengthen lower body muscles and build up stamina. It is advised to do fitness walking and stair climbing. It is recommended to start with ten minutes every day and then gradually increases the time. Try to do it at least five times a week.

Swimming
Swimming is considered as a fountain of youth and no doubt it helps to increase mobility of joints and strengthen them. When you swim there is less stress on the joints. You should start slowly then gradually increasing the swimming time. Here it is important to note that swimming speed and distance does not matter but the time is spent to improve the mobility of joints. Make a schedule of 15 minutes for two days in a week. Then gradually go for 30-45 minutes.

Stretching
Shoulders: Shoulder movements include placing hands by your side then roll shoulders in backward direction for 30 seconds then forward direction for 30 seconds.

Wrists: Roll your wrist by making a fist in clockwise and anti-clockwise directions for 30 second.

Back and Hamstrings: This exercise is done by sitting on the floor with your legs straight. Then reach forward towards your toe. Touch it and hold it for about 15 seconds and try to do it three times.

3) Weight

Obesity increases the risk of gout as discussed in earlier chapters, as it increases uric acid levels in the body and increases the risk of developing gout. So in other words, losing weight to a normal level would decrease uric acid levels in the body and its risk of developing gout. By reducing weight it is a lot easier to prevent future attacks. As compared with a person with an ideal body weight, an obese persob is four times more likely to develop gout in his lifetime. The physician should encourage weight loss in obese individuals to lower uric acid levels.

The physician must suggest diet plans and also the risks associated with them. Cutting back on fat is very important for gout patients. The body's ability to eliminate uric acid is reduced by saturated fat in the diet. Use of plant based proteins such as legumes and beans or dairy products low in fat would help to achieve the desired goals. As food rich in high fat content are often linked with obesity and ultimately with gout.

Take whole grains, fruits and vegetables in the diet. Don't get tempted by any crash diet, as rapid loss can trigger gout attacks and more complications. Here, a slow and steady logic will work. So ask your physician about it in detail and start making small changes in your diet which will sustain later in the long run.

4) Regular Checkup

It is recommended to get your uric acid levels checked every six months and make sure the level is below 6mg/dl.

5) Alcohol Consumption

Alcohol consumption and its relation with gout is centuries old. Alcohol increases uric acid in the body by formation of lactate due to excess hydrogen ions formed during alcohol oxidation. It also dehydrates the body, which in turn increases uric acid load in the body.
Two drinks per day are considered safe but in order to get rid of the disease one must abandon the use of alcohol completely.
Wine is not considered as much harmful as beer because beer not only contains alcohol but also rich in purine.

6) Fructose

Fructose is not only present in highly processed foods and soft drinks but also in many fruits and fruit juices. So in that case, a gout patient must pay attention to the daily fructose intake in the diet. It is recommended not to consume more than 25mg of fructose daily. Watch out for the fruits, fruit juices, processed foods, cereals, cookies and beverages that contain high fructose content. It should be noted that not all the sugars are same. Only fructose is capable of raising uric acid levels in the body within hours of ingestion. Research reveals that many soft drinks contain 58% fructose.

The leading soft drinks among them are Coca Cola, Pepsi and Sprite, which contain 68% fructose. These evil high fructose corn syrups contain a huge amount of fructose, which is 20 times sweeter than table sugar. Therefore it is absorbed immediately in the blood and directly goes to the liver. Therefore cutting down on these soft drinks is very important for maintaining normal levels of uric acid in the body. However, our prime goal is to prevent the increase of uric acid levels in the body and prevent obesity. Sugar is as addictive as cocaine as claimed by many researchers, a great deal of calories comes from sugar. It not only put us at a risk of gout but obesity and tooth decay as well.

7) Cutting out the stress in your life

Emotional pain and stress is found to be the root cause of many problems, especially gout. Studies reveal that stress triggers a painful gout attack in many patients. Although it is not possible to completely remove stress from life, there are ways to minimize it. Meditation and deep relaxation like yoga will help.

Key Points to Remember

So by taking the above mentioned precautions and changes in daily life, one can definitely beat gout.

- Exercising daily and reducing weight would help.
- Besides limiting red meat and food rich in purine content, enjoy a modest seafood or vegetable rich diet to purify and cleanse the body.
- Include skim milk and yogurt in the diet as a part of low fat dairy products.
- Take nuts, seeds and salads as a part of snacks.
- Avoid beer and liquor, as they are linked with triggering gout attack.
- Last but not the least, takes Vitamin C in the form of papaya, cherries and supplements.
- Make a special appointment with your doctor, dietitian and pharmacist. Ask them before making any sudden changes in the diet. Consult with them for the best diets and appropriate diet plans. You don't have to make drastic changes but go on making small changes then sustain them as long-terms plan. So work with your doctor and dietitian and see what works best in your favor

Chapter 10: Managing Gout and Coping With Gout

If you or someone that you care about has been diagnosed with gout, it can feel as if your world is shifting. You have been diagnosed with a possibly debilitating disease that will give you a severe amount of paint. You may feel as if your life is shifting out of control or that there is nothing that you can do.

While it is true that gout is a chronic condition, you must remember that you are not helpless. There is plenty of information out there when you are looking for a diet for gout, for home remedies for gout or for foods that cause gout.

Even if you are already receiving plenty of medical help and advice, you will always be ahead of the game if you are willing to be proactive about your care. Looking up gout home remedies, gout diets and what gout is caused by is something that can help you feel empowered. Whether you want to know more about gout causes and symptoms or you are on the hunt for a gout natural treatment that works for you, start your search today!

1) Gout Journaling

When it comes to looking at gout diet restrictions and trying to find the best gout treatment for you, it is very easy to start to get confused. You may be wondering whether that last natural gout remedy that you tried was really effective, or whether symptoms of the gout treatment you last tried were different than they were before.

As with any medical issue, keeping track of things like your day-to-day health and the medications and herbal gout remedies that you were considering can be difficult. There is a lot to remember, and remedies for gout pain can be quite diverse. As you proceed, you may find that there is no perfect remedy for gout pain, but instead you can create a perfect solution for your own needs.

As the doctors keep telling us, every person is different. No matter what you see on commercials, there is no one-size-fits-all solution when it comes to a problem like gout. Gout affects people in different ways and with different types of severity, and you never know when a solution is going to work for you.

With this in mind, a health journal is something that can be very helpful for you. A health journal is something that you can use to keep track of the gout symptoms and treatment plans that you have tried, a particular food to avoid, or the gout home remedy that you were considering. As you may have noticed, gout food to be avoided by one person is food that can be easily eaten by another.

To make a journal that you can carry around with you, simply pick a notebook from the store and clip a pen to it. Date the page, and write down anything that is pertinent to your condition. Some people take their notes in a very free-form way, while others prefer to answer the same questions over and over again.

For example, a list of questions for your gout health journal might include:

* Am I suffering from gout pain today?

* If I am suffering from gout pain, what is its intensity? (You may choose to rate the intensity of the pain from 1 to 10, just to give yourself an idea of whether the pain is increasing or decreasing over a certain span of time.

* What have I eaten today?

* Am I on my period?

*How much water have I drunk today?

*What medications have I taken today?

*What was my level of physical activity today?

These questions are just designed to get you started. You can answer them as completely and as detailed a fashion as you like. You are creating a record for your own use, though you may find that it is helpful to refer to this record when you are dealing with your doctor as well.

You may also find that there are apps for your Smartphone that will help you to keep track. There are several apps that tell you how much purine is in the food that you eat, and there are many general health apps out there that will tell you how much you have eaten in general and how healthy you are on a given day.

Apps tend to be a little less precise than keeping track of your condition on your own, however, so consider keeping a few notes of your own.

While keeping a journal might feel a little demanding or tedious at first, you will quickly find that in no time at all, it can make a huge difference to how you are looking at your health.

A big reason to try the gout journal is to simply remark on your food. Because many of us are so busy, it is often a lot of trouble to think about what we eat. We run to the fast food place around the corner, or we don't think about the snacks that we are currently consuming.

A food journal forces you to record everything that you eat, and if you know that you need to make the entry, you might find yourself pausing to think.

On top of that, a good health journal will also ensure that you record what treatments you have started and when they began. For example, a journal will help you figure out when you started the type of medication or when you began a treatment. In many cases, the treatments that you began will only begin to take effect slowly. Without a clear idea of when you began them, you might begin to grow impatient when it really takes several weeks to work, or you might continue a treatment that doesn't work for you believing that it will take more time.

A gout journal can go a long way towards teaching you more about how you are doing. It makes you stop to reflect what is going on with your body, and it makes you much more aware of how you feel.

Remember that a gout journal can be whatever it needs to be. While plenty of people prefer to have it in a physical form that they can carry around with them, other people prefer it to be an app that they fill out on their tablet or their Smartphone. Others prefer a middle of the road approach where they type all of their data into a document on their computer. If you decide to type your information into a document, consider getting a cloud-based archival service, so you have access to your document no matter what machine you happen to be on.

2) Be Patient

Remember that any treatment or diet that you use to treat gout should not have instant results. Even NSAIDs, which work to bring down inflammation and swelling, can take some time to work to their full efficiency.

Nothing is fixed overnight, and as with any other individualistic problem, you will discover that it might take you some time to get where you need to be.

Do not be discouraged when you are dealing with yet another gout attack. It can be painful to remember that this is a chronic condition, but the truth is that you will see some improvement with some diligent effort. You may feel as if you are helpless in the face of the pain, but the truth is that you do have some power over it.

It might take you weeks or even months to get a really good grip on what works for you, but once you have it, you will be in a much better place.

One of the worst things about the first few gout attacks is that you do not know what is going on. You are in a great deal of pain, and you may feel afraid as to what is going on in your body. This can make your situation seem even worse.

3) Support

When people think about treatment for gout, they often think solely in terms of methods to relieve pain. Given the fact that pain is such a significant part of this disorder, that makes sense, but there is an entire mental and emotional side to the disorder that needs to be addressed.

For example, you may feel that you brought the disorder on yourself. You may be ashamed of choices that you have made in the past or you may be worried as to what others think of you. It is essential to remember that gout is a disorder like any other. There is no one thing that causes it, and in many cases, it is often a perfect storm of attributes that bring it around.

Alternatively, you may be upset at the loss of mobility. If you are an active person, gout can put a serious kink in your plans. Depending on what you did before you suffered from gout, you may feel as if this condition has robbed you of important parts of your identity.

A diagnosis of gout can spin your life around. It is a chronic disorder, and it can affect you in many different ways. Do not be afraid to be sad, upset, or angry about it, and do not allow anyone to tell you how you should feel. While you should of course control your actions, you are entitled to feel how you want to feel about something that changes your life.

Look for support when you need it. Take advantage of your family and friends, and take them up on their offers. In many cases, it is too easy to feel as if you are a burden when the truth is that most of your friends would love to sit and hear about your remedy for gout or to find out what gout is caused by. They want to listen to you, they love you, and they care about you, so do not shut them out.

Be ready to give a little bit of education about gout as well. After all, gout is a bit obscure when it comes to portrayals in the media, and your friends will not know what foods cause gout or the signs and symptoms of arthritis pain. They will not know what foods to avoid with gout, which can make going over to a friend's place for a meal a little tricky, and they won't know about purines in food, all things that you have had to become an expert on.

Be willing to be an educator and to make sure that they know where you stand. Tell them about home remedies for gout pain or the brand new natural remedy for gout that you are currently invested in. A little bit of education can go a long way towards getting your friends to be the support group they want to be, so be willing to share with them and to help them understand where you are coming from.

4) Rest

One of the things that they do not often tell you about pain management is that pain is tiring. Even when you are not actively in pain, even when the pain itself is something that you can consider minor, you may find that you are simply tired all the time.

Firstly, think about why this is true. Gout causes pain that radiates from your joint to the rest of your body. That means that your body tenses in reaction to this pain. Constant tension throughout your frame is something that can leave you feeling exhausted!

When you are always tensed up, it does not matter what you know about foods causing gout or what causes gout. All that matters is that pain is radiating through your joint, causing your whole body to tense. The gout in foot symptoms that you might be suffering from are causing your body to stiffen up, and hold itself tense, and that is why a good gout remedy treatment will always include some kind of pain management.

Even when you are eating well and aware of what foods to avoid for gout, you will discover that you are getting tired. A gout attack makes your muscles tense up tightly, and when this happens, you will find yourself stressed out and exhausted.

Make sure that you account for this pain when you are having a rough time. If you feel a gout attack coming on, or you are recovering from one, you should remember that you are going to be tired. This means that you should be prepared to spend some time recuperating.

If at all possible, go to bed early. It is usually better to go to bed early and to wake up at your normal time rather than to simply stay up late and sleep in. This keeps your circadian rhythm on track, and it prevents you from staying up late when you are recovered.

Some people have a rough time sleeping if they are in pain, so consult your doctor about things like painkillers and sleep aids that are designed to be taken right before bed. Some people like to use medication to help them get to sleep, while others prefer to rely on natural methods, like warm almond milk and meditation.

If you want to take a natural approach to getting to sleep, the best thing that you can do is to create a wind-down routine. Half an hour before you actually go to bed to sleep, turn down the lights. Take a warm shower so that you are feeling relaxed, and consider eating something relatively light but full of protein.

Keep the room as quiet as you can, and simply let your mind drift. If you want to read before you to go sleep, do it in a chair rather than in the bed. If you can make sure that the bed is associated only with sleeping, you will be able to drift off much easier.

Before you go to sleep, take off your watch. Some people find that they are constantly checking the time as they sleep. They are either worried that they have to be up too soon, or they are concerned with how little sleep that they are getting. If any of this is the case for you, remove the watch, triple check your alarm if you need to, and put away this distraction.

Remember that sleep is when your body has time to heal from the problems that have been affecting it through the day. If your gout pain is preventing you from sleeping, it will only get worse. Some people manage to reduce their sleep until they are forced to fall asleep and then to build up to a full's night of rest in a short while, but this is something that can take time and effort.

When you are looking up herbal remedies to help you with sleep, consider valerian and St. John's wort, though you should check with your doctor to make sure that you are not getting anything that will interfere with your medication.

Another natural option for you to try is melatonin, which is often called the sleep hormone. Melatonin is a hormone that your body produces naturally, and it is what is used to send you to sleep. In many cases, the human body does not produce enough melatonin, and beyond that, disrupted lives and pain can reduce the production of melatonin even further. Pick up a bottle of melatonin at your local vitamin store, take it about half an hour before you mean to go to bed and see how well it works for you.

Remember that if you lose enough sleep, you can be as impaired as if you were drinking! Too little sleep takes a slow and gradual toll on you, and over time, it is something that will decrease your quality of life. Your mood starts to slip long before you think it does, your functionality goes way down, and you will discover that in no time at all, you are letting things slip that should not slip.

All of these symptoms are very serious, so when you are worried about them, or you are afraid they are affecting you, call your doctor.

If you are having pain on your foot, consider what you can do to keep your foot still. Some people pile up blankets on either side of the foot, creating a hollow. When your foot is placed in this hollow, it becomes much less inclined to roll around. If your foot is sensitive, stabilizing it can help you sleep through the night.

Remember to be gentle with yourself when you are looking at recovering from a gout attack. This is a paint that some have compared to childbirth, and you will discover that it can leave you feeling exhausted. Get the rest you need, and you will be on your feet much more quickly than you might be if you had pushed yourself.

5) Water And Plenty Of It!

We're told over and over again that water is good for gout, but what you might not know is why.

At the most basic level, water washes waste material out of your body. It allows your body to get rid of waste products from various metabolic functions, and it allows you to make sure that you do not have that waste causing harm in your body. You've heard the standard idea that everyone needs to drink at least eight glasses of water every day, but the truth of the matter is that in general, the more water you drink the better!

When you drink enough water, you are creating a way for your body to get rid of such things as the uric acid, which builds up and causes the crystals to form in your blood. When you keep your system well hydrated, you are creating a situation where you are keeping your uric acid levels as low as possible.

While some people do just fine when they are told to drink more water, it can be a little troublesome for people who never drank all that much water in the first place. As a matter of fact, most of us go through our lives being vaguely dehydrated without ever even knowing it!

How can you make sure that you get the water that you need? The right amount of water for you is a personal thing. You might choose to stick with the common eight glasses of water a day rule, because that will tend to get more water into you than not, but if you have a little more time, it is worth listening to the new scientific wisdom.

According to scientists today, to get the best use out of the water that you drink, take your body weight in pounds and divide that number in half. That number, in ounces, is how much water you should drink.

Take a moment to think about when and where you get your water. Some people drink their water with meals, but for the best results, you should consider drinking your water about an hour before you eat. This prevents the food from soaking up the water and carrying it out of your system before you can take advantage of it.

Consider getting a drink of water part of your daily routine. Get up and drink a glass of water, and then make sure that you have a tall glass whenever you take a break during the day. On top of that, consider having a glass of water a little bit after you work out or a few hours before lunch.

When you are thinking about how you can move forward towards drinking more water, consider carrying a water bottle around with you. A water bottle is a constant reminder that you should be drinking more, and if you want to make the water more interesting, you can add a little bit of flavoring, like with a squirt of lemon juice.

Remember that the best thing to drink is pure water. While things like sodas and teas are quite tasty, they are also diuretics. They encourage the water to leave your system sooner than it should, and with regards to gout, that is the last thing that you want.

Try to drink water whenever it is offered. When you are at a restaurant, ask for water, and when you pass a water fountain, take a drink. There are many great benefits for getting more water in your system anyway, so take the time to make sure that you are taking care of this basic gout attack preventative.

One important note to remember is that if you are taking any medication for your kidneys or if you are on any kind of diuretic, as people often are for their high blood pressure, contact your doctor about how much water you should be drinking.

6) Reduce Stress

Many people note that stress is something that brings on a gout attack. Sometimes, it is stress over work, and other times, it is stress over a family member or a romantic entanglement, but one moment, the person is frustrated about something, and in the next moment, they are dealing with sharp pains in their feet! Stress is something that can weaken your body's immune system and prevent it from fighting off gout attacks as effectively as it should. Stress is something that can take almost any situation and make it worse, and when you are dealing with something that comes and goes like a gout attack, you will find that it is time to see what kind of stressors you can remove from your life.

When it comes to how to treat gout, there is just so much information out there. Between natural remedies for arthritis, learning about purine foods and considering a uric acid diet, it can be hard to stay cheerful. As you contemplate a low purine diet and inform your family about your diet restrictions, you may start to feel a little run down.

This is exactly the kind of environment that can make stress much worse, and when you are looking to keep yourself healthy, that's when stress can attack.

At the most basic level, stress is a fight or flight experience. It is designed to help us fight off attacks from people who would do us harm, and it can also make sure that we get away if we decide to run. However, stress and adrenaline, the chemical that enables us to do these things, do not have the same applications as they once did. We can no longer run away from a fraught meeting with a family member, and we cannot simply punch a customer who is being annoying, even if we wish we could.

Instead, the stress builds up and builds up, and if we don't let it out, it starts to manifest in unhealthy ways. Some side effects of stress include panic attacks, anxiety, hives, constant fatigue and short tempers. In the case of gout, stress can actually induce a gout attack.

When you first look at it, calming down the stress in your life feels like a huge task. Often, most of the things that are stressing you out do not have easy answers. If they did, you wouldn't be stressed out about them! However, you will find that it is essential for you to both identify the type of stress you are experiencing and then to figure out how to calm your reaction to it.

When you are trying to identify the source of your stress, think about when you feel the most frustrated or the most helpless. Too many people think that there must only be one thing that is causing them stress, when the truth of the matter is that it is likely to be several different things.

Think about what you feel throughout the day. Sometimes, the thing that is causing you stress is such an every-day occurrence that it startles you to realize that you are harboring such frustrated emotions so often.

If you are feeling stumped when it comes to sources of your stress, start keeping a journal and note down your feelings throughout the day. One way to organize this is to divide the page into two columns. Label the column on the left "Things That Happened," and label the column on the right "How I Felt." If you start to fill this out truthfully, you will soon discover the source of your stress.

Once you have figured out why you are feeling stressed, you need to think about what to do. Stress is an emotion that leaves you feeling tired and drained, but it is not because you have done something. Instead, it is frequently because you were not able to do something.

One saying goes that you should control what you can control, and do your best to work around the rest. If you are constantly pounding your head against something that cannot be changed, you are not going to feel better. Accept that some things are beyond your power and move on. Although you might fear that this is too much like giving up, the truth is that it simply means that you are preserving your energy for a better purpose.

Create a plan of action. If you are someone who thrives with lists and rules, you will quickly discover that they can make you feel better about things that are stressing you out. Think about the problems that are frustrating you at this moment, and think about what you can do about them.

If there are things that you cannot change, you should find out how you can make it so that they do not bother you so much. For example, if you have a family member who is behaving poorly, think about a way to make sure that you stay away from them until they improve or the circumstances change.

There are many methods that are ideal for making sure that stress leaves your body, and many of them are great for gout as well. Check the section below for exercise and how to do it in a way that will not hurt you, but also consider things that will smooth away some of the ragged edges of the day. You may know all about low purine recipes, gout diet plans and gout symptoms treatment, but do you also know how to take care of yourself.

When you are just getting used to the symptoms for gout and learning what gout symptoms are, you may have forgotten about some of the things that usually relax you. If reading that made you think that it's been a while since you've watched a movie or did some knitting, pick it up again. Our brains love patterns and even if you are suffering from gout symptoms, you can enjoy them. Meditation is a great choice for getting stress relief from gout, and though you might associate it with highly spiritual people, it is in fact an exercise that you can use in your day-to-day life to center yourself. Meditation can last anywhere from a few minutes to a few hours, and when you are getting started, look for meditation tracks on streaming sites like YouTube. Get the track started, and simply meditate as long as it takes to finish the track.

To start meditating, simply sit in a comfortable way that will not allow you to fall asleep. Let your eyes drift shut, and concentrate on your breathing. When you first start meditating, thoughts will drift in and out. Let your mind think about them, but do not dwell on them. Think of your mind as a river or a stream. Focus on one segment, and just as things come in, let them drift away.

Empty your mind, slow your breathing, and for the length of the track, just exist. You have many things going on in your life, not in the least of which is gout, but for the moment, you do not have to think about them. You are giving yourself a break. You will take up your responsibilities in five, ten, or thirty minutes, but as you exist right now, you do not need to think about anything at all. Meditation is a great way to reduce stress, and in that way, you can use it to prevent gout attacks.

When you are looking for a more active way to relax, you might consider volunteer work. Even if you are working under the assumption that you will have bad days with your gout, and even when you are concerned about what you can really handle, there are some fantastic activities that are perfect for you.

Remember that while gout can take some things away from you, it cannot take away the person that you really are. The issues with gout that you have do not change what your mind and your spirit are like. If you are not worried too much about decreased mobility and you are relatively healthy, why not volunteer with your local park service? If you love kids, consider joining a free day care program, and if you have a knack for computers, offer to do some coding for the local non-profit of your choice!

7) Exercise

Think about starting an exercise regimen that you really love. Exercise creates a situation where stress can leave your body and where you can make sure that you are giving your body the movement that it needs.

Before you start exercise, however, it is important to speak to a doctor. This is especially true if you have not exercised in any sort of concentrated way in the last few years. People like to say that exercise is something that everyone should do, but the truth is that not everyone should do it in the same way. If you have undiagnosed herniated disks, for example, exercise that does not take them into account can actually leave you bedridden and in worse shape than you started out.

If you are overweight, there is a chance that a doctor will okay you for exercise without much of an exam or a talk. This is a sign that the doctor is not seeing beyond your weight, and it is also a sign that you need a new doctor! Exercise creates stress in the body, and if you do not know what you are doing, it can actually create chronic issues that will be with you for years, if not decades. Talk with your doctor about a thorough physical, any physical issues that might have you concerned, and which exercises might be right for you. Someone who is relatively healthy will likely do fine with a heavy cardio workout, while someone with weaker or damaged joints might need to stick to low-impact exercises like water aerobics or yoga.

Remember that exercise is something that needs to suit you. Do not push yourself to do a kind of exercise that frustrates or annoys you. While no pain, no gain is widely dismissed as a poor way to get in shape or treat your body, it cannot be denied that exercise is an investment in time, and often in money.

Think about your life and first consider where exercise can fit in. While it has some great health benefits, the amount of stress that is caused when exercising can be significant. For example, think about whether you want to exercise before or after work, with friends or completely on your own, and how much money you can spend on it. Your exercise needs to fit into your life. It should not be a cause of stress!

Remember that you will miss a workout from time to time. The key is to make sure that you make each missed workout an incident rather than a trend. Plenty of people miss workouts here and there, so do not feel demoralized if you do too.

What kind of exercise appeals to you? When it comes to dealing with gout, nearly any kind will do. A gout attack can leave you unable to workout in some ways, but there are still exercises that you can do to stay limber. During a gout attack, you need to take care of yourself, but otherwise, the rest of the time, exercise can often be conducted normally.

Try to find a type of physical activity that you can look forward to. If you are someone who is deeply interested in time outside, by yourself, think about going for solitary runs in the park. If you love the feeling of camaraderie and you have a performing streak, think about joining a dance troupe. There are plenty of great ways for you to get exercise out there.

If you love zombie movies, pick up a Smartphone app that shows you how to get in shape for the zombie apocalypse, and if you are worried about people seeing you and making fun of you, pick up a jump rope and work out at home.

8) The RICE Method

If you have ever been around people who treat or receive sports injuries, you have likely heard about the RICE method of treating sports injuries. One thing that you may not know, however, is that it is also a great way to treat the affected area before, during, and after gout attacks. While the cause of gout is not always known, and while gout diet foods have changed as our understanding of the condition has gotten better and better, the RICE method, in one form or another, has been used consistently. RICE is an acronym that stands for Rest, Ice, Compress, and Elevate.

Rest is obvious, and when you are looking over a gout diet menu and deliberating between gout treatments, you might not be inclined to do anything but rest, but this can serve as a reminder. Gout attacks take a lot out of you, so as you go over your gout diet list one more time, get some rest.

Ice is used to cool the inflammation around the area and it can also be used to bring down swelling in the affected location. Ice is also used to numb the area, meaning that as you work on your gout symptoms diet, you will be able to reduce the pain as well. Be careful with ice as it is possible to overdo it, but in general, if you wrap the ice in a thin towel, you will be fine. If you do not have ice to hand, you can simply use a frozen television dinner or other frozen boxes to cool your inflammation.

It is important to remember that the use of ice in gout treatment is somewhat controversial. Some people adore the use of ice to treat their gout attacks, while other people shudder to think of the cold on flesh that is that sensitive.

Experiment with it to see how you find it to work for you. You may be able to take some cold, you might love having it on your painful area, or you might not like it at all. It is always worth remembering that every home treatment for gout is different, and what works for someone else might not always work for you.

To compress an area affected by gout, you can use a standard bandage or you can simply do it much more gently with a long towel or length of fabric. One great thing to do is to heat a towel in the microwave and to use it to gently wrap the area. Do not wrap the area too tightly. A tight wrap is intended to help you move around, and if you have a gout attack, you want to avoid that as much as possible. Heat a towel very lightly in the microwave, wrap it around your foot or ankle, and settle in to look over your gout diet list.

Finally, elevate the affected limb. It sounds almost cartoonish, but you can actually drain the blood from the inflamed area by getting gravity on your side. Use a cushion or a pillow to prop your leg up. Some people even do this when they sleep.

The RICE method is definitely something that should be included in your gout self-care regimen, right up there with gout herbal remedies and lists of gout diet foods to avoid.

9) Heat

When it comes to home remedies for gout treatment, heat is one of the things that often gets brought up, but some people find that its use is controversial. They say that heat only makes the area more inflamed and does no good at all. While cold is often recommended to relieve pain, it is important to remember that heat serves a different purpose.

The addition of heat can bring more oxygen to a wound, helping it to heal more quickly. This means that heat is often traded off with cold when it comes to treating gout.

As any gout remedy report will tell you, exercise is important. However, if you are stiff from a recent gout attack, it is not safe for you to immediately jump into your aerobics program! This is where heat can come in. Use heat to loosen up the affected area before you start your exercise routine, and then afterwards consider icing it to calm down the area. Remember that any really severe gout attack means that you should be very careful with yourself, just as you know to be careful about gout and foods to avoid.

Be very careful with heat, as some people find that its use makes the area worse. Other people enjoy the pain relief that they get from the heat, but find that they need to drink a lot more water to cope with the dehydrating effect of the heat.

Do not use extreme heat of any sort to treat gout; keep it mild.

10) Finding a Herbal Remedy for Gout

When it comes to looking up gout remedies, natural options are sure to come up. As a matter of fact, there are many natural remedies for gout, and herbal options are often milder and less severe in terms of side effects than drugs that you would get over the counter or from the doctor.

As you look up natural treatments for gout, you will find that most of the herbs that are recommended for natural treatment of gout all have a certain factor in common. They are all used to treat inflammation of the joints. Virtually any herb that is commonly used to treat inflammation can be used to treat gout. As you consider your gout treatment, natural remedies can play a big part in how you go about it.

As you look into gout foods, one of the best things that you can do is to look into supplements that are made from foods that are high in anti-oxidants. Anti-oxidants work to remove inflammation from your body, and some of the most effective ones include blueberry, bilberry, rapeseed, and pineapple supplements. Bilberry and pineapple are especially great options to consider when you are looking at gout treatments that are more natural. Bilberry is rich in anthocyanin, which are designed to help your body direct its blood flow. This is an excellent thing in a gout attack, where blood flow is slowed in the affected area. Pineapple supplements are rich in bromelain, a substance that helps the body to reduce the amount of uric acid in the blood.

Another great herbal remedy to try when you are looking at figuring out how to create a good treatment for gout is devil's claw. Devil's claw is a distinctively shaped herb that is also often called the unicorn plan. It is available in a dried, powdered capsule form, making it easy to ingest, and it does several things to help with gout. It is a powerful anti-inflammatory, and it is also thought to lower the levels of uric acid in the body.

This herbal remedy is typically taken when the first twinges of a gout attack start, and people speak enthusiastically about it bringing down the length of a gout attack from weeks down to mere days. When you are looking at gout treatments, natural remedies might be more effective than you thought. Devil's claw is easy to find at any reasonably stocked vitamin or alternative health store, and it is definitely worth a shot.

As you consider your gout treatment, natural methods can show you the way. The right treatment for gout varies from person to person, but as you learn more about the causes of gout, you can also learn a lot about gout home remedies for pain treatment.

11) Accept the Fact that Gout Attacks Will Just Happen

Even people with excellent management techniques and a thorough idea of what they are doing are going to have gout attacks. Remember that gout is a chronic condition and that no matter what you do about it, it will affect your life. No matter how much you know about foods for gout diet, what to eat for gout diet or gout treatment diet home remedies, there are going to be days where you find yourself dealing with gout attacks.

Some people get very demoralized when they feel as though they have done everything right, and they still get gout attacks. The truth is that you can be on the most rigorous purine diet for gout treatment and you can be on great medication for gout treatment, and you might still have an attack.

This does not mean that you should give up all hope of stopping a gout attack! It only means that you are not perfect and that your body simply functions in a way that is less than desirable. Do not fault yourself for something you can't control.

12) Manage Your Pain

If you are aware of the right gout diet for you, and if you are being otherwise very careful, you might start to get a little worried about the pain. You may begin to feel that the pain is your fault, or that you can tough it out.

Pain is not a punishment, it is not something that you need to endure, and whether you bear it quietly or loudly, it comes to the same thing. Pain is simply your body telling you that there is something wrong.

Gout attacks bring pain with them, and as any medical professional will tell you, pain is not a mild thing. It is a serious condition that can make your life very hard. It can stop you from doing things that you want to do, and it can make you feel extremely vulnerable.

Do not think that you have to bear pain in silence. Pain does not get better unless you do something to stop it, so be aware of your pain and advocate for yourself. If your medication is not working to control your pain, talk to your doctor. If a certain type of exercise is aggravating your pain, stop and find an alternative option.

Simply enduring pain silently is something that we are taught is a virtue, but the truth is that it does not serve us well.

If you are in pain, the best thing that you can do is to treat it or find a way to mitigate it.

No one is saying that you should expect the pain to go away entirely. Just be aware that there is a space between no pain at all and searing agony. Do not be afraid to look for pain management solutions.

You get no credit and no gain from staying silent, so speak up!

13) Regular Doctor Visits

If you have a serious case of gout, the truth is that the doctor is going to want to see you on a regular basis. If you were relatively healthy before, you may have managed to skip regular visits routinely.

However, the thing to remember is that knowing what foods you should avoid if you have gout and gout diet causes are just the tip of the iceberg. When it comes to good gout medication, treatment involves getting yourself to a professional.

Remember that the levels of uric acid in your blood should be regularly monitored, and that your doctor is the only one who can perform the tests. Learning what gout foods to eat and avoid is also something that your doctor can help you with.

Speak with your doctor about how often they want to see you. Depending on the case and depending on what your needs are, they may be fine seeing you once a year, but some want to see you every six months or even more often.

One of the best things that you can do when you are looking at staying healthy while dealing with gout is to consult with professionals regularly. They are the ones that can tell you when a change is just a normal thing and when it is something to be seriously worried about, and they can also help you to figure out what you need to change.

Try to make sure that you see going to the doctor as a necessary thing, rather than something that you can just do or avoid as you please!

14) Learning to Say No

One thing that is going to surprise you, especially if you have never had to deal with any sort of eating restriction before, is how pushy people can get about food!

It takes a lot of time and effort for you to figure out what not to eat for gout and to look into food that causes gout, and that's after you've weeded out the pseudo gout diet plans out there that get in the way!

After you've spent all this time gathering the knowledge that will keep you healthy, it is entirely fair for you to get irritable with all the people who say "but just this once won't hurt!" or "you just need to try this steak, it'll be fine!'

Food is one of the ways that we make others feel included, whether we understand that or not, and sometimes, it seems that others do not care about what gout is and the symptoms associated with it, they just want to make sure that you try their liver and onion dish!

Be very firm with people, and remind them gently that you are dealing with a medical disorder. This is not something that they have a right to pressure you over, especially if they are the kind of people who want to push the latest homeopathic gout treatment or pseudo gout treatment onto your lap. If they get aggressive, remember that you have a right to look after your health, and that you are the person in charge of what you put into your mouth!

This is not to say that you will not be tempted. Sometimes, people will just want to go to the sushi place where all you can really have is cucumber roll, and sometimes, you will go to a family dinner where all you can eat are the whole-wheat bread rolls.

This can be a tricky situation to deal with, but one thing that you can do is to pre-eat. Before you go, eat a full meal of something that you have prepared for yourself, and that you know is safe. When you get to the event itself, you can simply eat appetizers or anything else that is safe.

When you are dealing with a trip, do your best to pre-plan. Look over menus for fast food places that will be en route. Places that prepare personalized sandwiches are your best bet for staying safe, as is any place that has a good menu for vegetarian cuisine. If someone else is planning the trip, make sure that they are aware of your needs.

Remember that you should also consider what to do at social drinking situations. Sometimes, it's hard to be denied your favorite drinks when everyone else around you is having a good time. One way to feel a little better about this is to volunteer to be the designated driver. You might also bring up the situation with a close friend and ask if they want to keep it limited with you when your friend group goes out.

Saying no to anything can be tough, especially when people are asking about things that you previously would have been delighted to accept. Remember that you are doing what you are doing for your health, and stick to your guns!

15) Take a Footbath

As you learn more about gout remedies at home and as you reach out to look for the gout cure treatment that will work for you, it might be a good idea to start taking footbaths, or simply learning to submerge any affected part in hot water. Remember that using heat is a bit controversial in the gout community, but there are enough people who get good results from it for you to give it a try!

As you are learning what foods to avoid when you have gout, also think about the kind of home care treatments you can do. A footbath is a simple thing, and when you are dealing with a gout attack, you will find that it can make a huge difference to how you are moving forward.

To take a footbath, you simply need a foot basin from the local drug store. Just about any bucket or container will do, but it is a good idea to make sure that your feet have enough space and enough room so that you can stretch out and feel really comfortable.

Fill the foot basin with enough hot water so that you can completely submerge your feet, and simply sit and soak in the luxury for a little while. You can stay in for just five minutes if you want some instant relief, or you can simply use the footbath for an hour or so, adding warm water as the water cools down.

While you can certainly leave the footbath plain, there are a number of different things you can add into the mix. For example, some people find that adding a few teaspoons of Epsom salts to the water can help reduce swelling and bring about pain relief, while other people swear by adding a few drops of their favorite essential oils, like lavender and citrus.

One of the interesting things about the uric acid crystals that cause gout is that they are soluble in heat. As a matter of fact, it only takes a few degrees above body temperature to make them dissolve somewhat. However, as the body lowers to the normal temperature, they will re-form.

Whether a warm water bath works for you or not is a personal thing. Some people enjoy instant relief from a footbath, while other people find that they do best when they keep the area at a steady room temperature.

If the footbath makes your foot feel worse instead of better, don't do it. Do not use a footbath where the water is simply too hot, and make sure that you dry your feet completely afterwards.

16) Gout and Acupuncture

When you are in a spot where you are interested in making sure that your gout gets better and you would like to try some alternatives to drugs, it is worth your while to try acupuncture. Acupuncture is a method used in Traditional Chinese Medication, and it is shown to have some excellent effects on both reducing the pain of gout attacks and reducing the frequency as well. Acupuncture relies on the insertion of very thin hollow needles into specific points on the back, arms and legs. In some cases, the practitioner might run small jolts of electricity through the needles in order to stimulate the muscles. Though it might look a little alarming, it is generally quite painless. Afterward, people report feeling a great deal more energetic and dealing with a great deal less pain.

When you go looking for an acupuncturist, remember that you can treat it in the same way as when you are looking for a doctor. Find out who is recommended, ask people in the community, and go in for a consultation rather than an appointment.

Talk with your acupuncturist and ask where they studied. If you get any sort of strange vibe from the office, back away and try another clinic. The truth is that, as with so many other decisions to be made about your health, this is all about your comfort level.

You will often need to strip down to your underwear when you are dealing with an acupuncturist, and if you wear a bra, you might be asked to remove it. If this makes you uncomfortable, bring a friend or ask the person performing the procedure if there is anything that they can do to work around it.

When you go in to speak with an acupuncturist, make sure that they know what you are going through and the kind of problems that you are hoping to relieve. There are many people who are interested in acupuncture for a variety of reasons, so be willing to be explicit.

Ask them what you can reasonably expect in terms of improvement, and be diligent in monitoring it for yourself. Some people find that acupuncture works very well for them, and others prefer to stick to their own methods.

Chapter 11: Inflammation in Gouty Arthritis

An increased inflammatory response is usually observed in almost all chronic illnesses. Therefore, it's considered as the root cause of many health problems. Many factors contribute to inflammation such as lifestyle, stress, lack of activity or exercise in daily routine and eating habits.

Consumption of food products and soft drinks rich in fat, purines and sugar content trigger an inflammatory response which is very difficult to control if not treated at the right time. In this chapter, we will explore the mechanism of inflammation in gout and its types in detail.

1) What is Inflammation?

Our body is exposed to a variety of potentially harmful chemicals and substances including trauma, infection, heat, cold and radiation. Inflammation is our body's self-defense mechanism, which activates in the presence of harmful or irritating substances in our body. It is a sign of healing which comes in the form of inflammation.

Our body is naturally trying to get rid of the harmful substances. The self-protection begins with the removal of injured or damaged cells, irritant or pathogens from the body and healing starts. Infection is caused by any bacteria, virus or fungi and our body protects itself and responds in the form of inflammation. It is a part of our immune system to protect our body.

First, there is irritation, which then develops into inflammation. Then the healing process of a body starts, followed by discharge of pus. We are born with innate immunity, which is naturally present in our body as a defense mechanism. Another is adaptive immunity, which is achieved after a vaccination or infection. Many chemical mediators, proteins, blood vessels and blood cells are involved in the process of inflammation. There are two types of inflammatory cells, which are phagocytic and non-phagocytic that perform phagocytosis. Phagocytic cells are polymorph nuclear leukocytes (PNL), which includes eosinophil, basophil, neutrophils and macrophages whereas non phagocytes are lymphocytes and plasma cells.

2) Why Does Inflammation Cause Pain?

Inflammation is characterized by pain, stiffness, discomfort and distress. It depends on the severity of pain. Sometimes it is constant and steady called an ache. It is supposed to be an individual experience and could be throbbing, pulsating or pinching in nature.

Besides acute and chronic it can also be:

Nociceptive pain
There are different receptors in our body that sense this kind of pain. Changes in temperature, vibration and stretch are sensed by these receptors. This pain is triggered by any external force and our nervous system and stimuli react to it. In contrary, non-nociceptive means the pain which is caused due to any internal factors.

Somatic pain
Somatic pain is a kind of nociceptive pain in which muscles, bones, joints and ligaments are affected. These receptors are prone to temperature, inflammation and vibration. Musculo-skeletal pain and muscle cramps are also kind of somatic pain.

Visceral pain

Visceral pain is felt in deep organs of the body such as heart, liver, kidney, bowels, spleen, uterus, ovaries and main body cavities. These receptors sense a lack of oxygen, inflammation and stretch in the body. It is very difficult to describe and detect visceral pain, as it is a very deep ache.

3) Types Of Inflammation

Inflammation is of two types; Acute and Chronic inflammation.

a) Acute inflammation

It is described as an early response to tissue damage which starts within seconds and last days or even a year. The main risk factors that contribute to acute inflammation are various chemicals, infection, burns, infarction and trauma. After this event the body's defense system activates and tries to remove the infective agent.

There are various chemical mediators which facilitate the process of acute inflammation.

These chemical mediators are released from;
a - Infective agent,
b - Parenchymal cells,
c - Endothelial cells,
d - Mast cells,
e - Tissue macrophages,
f - Fibroblasts,
g -Extracellular matrix.

These inflammatory mediators induce changes in blood vessels and create a vascular response. Blood flow is increased as a result of dilation of the arteries that supply blood to the affected part. Fluid and proteins move into interstitial spaces as capillaries get more permeable due to inflammation.

Migration of neutrophils and macrophages in the interstitial spaces takes place. As neutrophil contains tiny sacs which have enzymes to digest harmful pathogens in the cell. While macrophages also perform the similar function and engulf the harmful foreign particle. Neutrophils are our first defense mechanism and protect our body from harmful invaders. Their effective manipulation is our crucial interest as their over activity also triggers heart problem and autoimmune problems. You may notice that when there is a cut on the skin it turns into a pale red line, which shows immediately capillaries are filled with blood and migration of fluid and blood proteins in the spaces is taking place.

Vascular response
As a result of vascular response, vasodilation of arterioles, veins and capillaries takes place which results in hyperemia. Endothelial cells swell and retract resulting in endothelial permeability. This results in entry of fluid rich in protein and inflammatory cells in the affected area which slows down the circulation because the viscosity of blood is increased. There might be release of red blood cells if the blood vessels are damaged. Endothelial cells play an important role in this process, as it produces nitric oxide and prostacyclin. These two chemicals prevent platelet aggregation and cause vasodilation.

Exudation
Fibrinogen is converted into fibrin which limits and controls the speed of foreign invaders. The presence of Exudate is indicative of an increase in vascular permeability and increase in the protein content of the cell.

Phagocytosis
Neutrophils and macrophages are important phagocytic cells. Opsonins (complement components with immunoglobulins) combine with antigens and promote phagocytosis. This antigen/opsonin complex attaches itself on the receptor of phagocyte and forms phagosome.

This phagosome combines with lysosome and forms phagolysosome. This lysosomal content kills the antigen and neutrophils also die, contributing to tissue damage because of the release of lysosomal content.

Type of Acute Inflammatory Exudate

Exudates vary according to the affected part and the reason of the injury.

Suppurative or Prulent
Exudate is rich in neutrophils and forms pus. Here, necrosis occurs because of lysosomal enzymes and oxygen derived free radicals. It can occur in body cavity. It turns into abscess when it is formed in any deep tissue or organ.

Serous
White blood cell immigration takes place and thin fluid is formed e.g. blisters.

Fibrinous
In case of an underlying acute inflammation it is formed on surfaces of cavities.

Systemic Effects of Inflammation

Fever
Macrophages produce chemical mediators such as IL1, IL6 and TNF in response of acute inflammation. These mediators' help in the formation of prostaglandins in the hypothalamus of the brain. This facilitates the formation of neurotransmitters, which resets the body temperature.

Malaise
* Unpleasant feeling,
* Decreased appetite,
* Loss of hunger and pain,

* Tachycardia,
* Neutrophilia,
Neutrophil count increases because of IL1 and TNF release from macrophages. This also increases neutrophils in the bone marrow. The neutrophils released from bone marrow are immature.

Mediators of Acute inflammation
During an acute inflammation, a number of chemical substances are derived from cells, which enter via inflammatory exudates in the cell. They usually have a short life span and cause vasodilation and increase vascular permeability.

Mediators
Vasodilation
Vasodilation is caused by nitric oxide, histamine, bradykinin, prostaglandins, and platelet activating factor (PAF).
Neutrophil adhesion
IL-1, TNF-alpha, PAF, C5a, leukotrienes, and chemokines.
Increased Permeability
Histamine, C3a, C5a, bradykinin, leukotrienes, nitric oxide and PAF.
Fever
IL-1, TNF-alpha, prostaglandins
Pain
Prostaglandins, bradykinin,
Neutrophil chemotaxis
C5a, leukotriene, bacterial components and chemokines.
Tissue necrosis
lysosomal content and free radical.

Causes of Acute Inflammation

1) Infection Bacterial or viral infection
2) Immune Reactions e.g. Bee sting
3) Other stimuli e.g. Heart attack, trauma, radiation, burns, and foreign bodies.

Cardinal Signs of Inflammation

Calor (Heat)
There is more blood in the affected area, which makes it hot.

Rubor (Redness)
Vasodilation of blood vessels which causes redness.

Tumor (Edema)
Swelling cause by edema

Dolor (Pain)
Extreme sensation of pain due to the release of prostaglandins and kinins.

Functio laesa (Loss of function)
Immobility or loss of function

Outcomes of Acute inflammation

Here, three things matter: the affected tissue, the extent of damage and duration of damage. Phagocytosis of debris and macrophages drain to lymphoid tissues takes place. Neutrophils die and a specific response of the body is developed. Proliferation of Parenchymal cells takes place followed by scar tissue. This starts the initiation and progression of chronic inflammation. If not treated on time chronic abscess will form.

b) *Chronic inflammation*

When acute inflammation is not treated at the right time it passes on to another phase, which is chronic inflammation. Tissue damage occurs at the same time as while the body tries to heal itself. There is increased blood flow and capillary permeability. The prime purpose of this process is the removal of harmful pathogens from the body. Till the damaging chemical is removed this pain can persist for years.

Chronic inflammation is mediated by T lymphocytes and B lymphocytes, plasma cells and macrophages along with the presence of scar tissues and an acute inflammatory response. First neutrophils enter the infected tissue followed by macrophages and lymphocytes. Macrophages have a longer life span than neutrophils.

Features Of Chronic Inflammation

Cells

Lymphocytes
These are formed in the bone marrow and are supposed to have a long life span. They are found in many tissues and are attracted by various chemotactic factors. This activates T lymphocytes and B lymphocytes as a chronic inflammation response. T cells are the helper cells and secrete cytokines in the immune response. In contrast to B cells which differentiate in areas of lymphoid tissues.

Plasma cells
They produce antibodies in the cell.
Natural killer cells:
As the name implies they have the ability to kill cells, which appear harmful.

Macrophages
They are normally found in tissues and are derived from monocytes. They are attracted by chemotactic factors. Many factors, such as interferon gamma and bacterial toxins activate them. They secrete inflammatory mediators in immune response.

Variable Granulation tissue
They are involved in the repairing of the cell and cause scarring. They consist of thin walled blood vessels, macrophages, lymphocytes, chronic inflammatory cells and Fibroblasts, which participate in collagen production.

Mediators of Chronic inflammation

T-Lymphocytes
Interferon gamma, which activates macrophages.
Interleukin-2 which stimulates T lymphocytes proliferation in the cell

Macrophages
Chemotactic factors, mediators of tissue destruction, mediators of bacterial killings, cytokines, growth factors and lymphocytes activating factor.

Causes of Chronic Inflammation

- Exposure to irritants or infection in the body,
- Untreated acute inflammation such as otitis and rhinitis,
- Primary chronic inflammation,
- Autoimmune reactions such as rheumatoid arthritis, glomerulonephritis and multiple sclerosis.

4) Mechanism of Acute Attack in Gout

In gout, an innate immune system regulates the inflammatory response. It immediately responds to the inflammatory response in contrary to adaptive system, which relies on the formation of antibodies and lymphocytes. When the receptors of the innate immunity system recognize monosodium urate crystals, then a protein scaffolding forms inflammasome which leads to the entry of an enzyme which acts on pro IL-1 and converts it into its active form IL-1β. As soon this active form is released in extracellular space it initiates a series of inflammatory responses.

It is the point where the entry of neutrophils along with other inflammatory mediators occurs. In humans, there are both intra and extracellular sensors in the form of receptors referred to pattern recognition receptors (PPRs) referred and as pathogen associated molecular patterns (PAMPs) which differentiate between viral and microbial cells. Theses sensors are called danger associated molecular patterns (DAMPs) in case of uric acid crystals.

This causes an activation of the inflammasome NLRP3 which is associated with the inflammatory response of uric acid crystals. Many innate immunity receptors have been identified now, including toll like receptors (TLRs) and C type Lectin receptors in the plasma membrane, lysosomes, endosomes and endoplasmic reticulum. The cell cytosol also contains receptors including the retinoic -acid inducible -gene -I-like -helicases or RIG-I-Like receptors (RLRS). Another receptor called Nod (nucleotide oligomerization domain) like receptors (NLRS) are also present in the cytosol.

These receptors are much diversified in differentiating among microbes and monosodium urate crystals. In the case of gout, these receptors work along with innate immunity receptors which form inflammasome; a complex protein. NLRS forms a group of 20 innate immunity receptors in humans. NLRS can not only distinguish among microbes, bacteria, virus and fungi but also non microbial danger signals.

Inflammasome mediates conversion of pro IL-1β to IL-1β its active form. The NLRP3 and NLRC3 inflammasome members of NLR family are very beneficial for gout. In the inflammatory response, aspartic acid specific cysteine proteases plays an important role. The three inflammatory starters caspase-1, caspase-4, and caspase-5 helps in conversion of pro IL-1β to IL-1β active form.

Interleukin -1β and Interleukin-18

Interleukin-1 is an important cytokine that generates many other inflammatory cytokines like IL-6, arachidonic acid and chemokines. It has two forms IL-1α and IL-1β. Fever angiogenesis and proliferation of Fibroblasts are important attributes of IL-1α. It's a very important interleukin working on many sites, whereas, IL-18 is formed from macrophages and dendritic cells. It's one of the strongest pro inflammatory cytokine, which forms nitric oxide, chemokines and IFN-γ which is responsible to activate macrophages.

Intervention

Certain modifiable risks can be prevented by making small changes in ones life style. Management of chronic illness can be done by following these recommendations:

- Eat a balanced diet along with exercise,
- Whole grain food must be added in the diet,
- Physical activity increases dietary consumption so exercise is very important in daily routine,
- Fruits and vegetable intake must be higher,
- Consumption of fish, especially once in a week,
- Don't eat saturated fats, take fat free and low dairy products,
- Don't eat over processed foods,
- Cut down on sugar and soft drinks,
- Avoid alcohol,
- Don't smoke,
- Avoid mental stress,
- Supplements after consulting with a doctor will be beneficial to many patients.

Inflammation is our body's self-defense to remove harmful and obnoxious organisms from the body. This is not only the root cause of gout but also diseases like insulin resistance, heart problems and many other chronic illnesses. Many phyto-chemicals are beneficial in such conditions.

There are many foods that alter the inflammatory response in our body. Foods rich in saturated fats and sugar also trigger inflammation. C reactive protein (CRP) is an important clinical bio marker for detection of inflammation. It's a protein synthesized in the liver and used as a clinical marker for inflammation besides measurement of erythrocytes sedimentation rate (ESR) and white blood cell count. High ESR rate and low blood cell count and low albumin levels are markers of inflammation. These tests are sometimes nonspecific and may end up in altered results.

Cytokine tests are not recommended, as they are not helpful in identifying the root of inflammation. Maintaining an ideal body weight is crucial. A lot of researchers have revealed that there are a lot of exercising techniques that reduces acute and chronic inflammation in the body. Reduction in numbers of cytokines is observed after following a healthy routine with exercise.

Chapter 12: Significance of Nutrition & Diet in Gout

1) Primary Care Benefits

Health departments in many countries provide general nutritional education under a "Public Health Care" program. Such programs are designed to educate the general public about the health benefits of a balanced diet and nutritional supplements. Surely, there are certain steps that must be carried out as primary care throughout life, especially during severe illnesses. Undoubtedly, the role of proper eating and anti-inflammatory diet in all types of arthritis, including gout, is inevitable. In fact, the role of diet in any medical complication is significant to control and reduce problematic symptoms.

2) Naturopathic Approach to Treat Gout

Naturopathic treatment is basically targeted to treat diseases like gout with holistic and nontoxic approaches with a substantial emphasis on disease prevention and optimizing wellbeing. Naturopathic medicine has proved to be helpful to treat several severe illnesses including cancer, thyroid problems, depression, fatigue, anxiety, asthma, digestive complaints, skin complaints, menstrual irregularities, chronic infections, autoimmune diseases, and gout.

3) Role of Calcium & Vitamin D in Mitigating Excellent Bone & Joint Health in Gout Patients

Nutritional supplementation can play a significant role in coping with gout symptoms.

It is necessary to take vital minerals from an exogenous source apart from diet. Calcium & Vitamin D are great sources to provide strength to bones and joints, and keep them healthy.

Deficiency of calcium within the body leads to deformation of bones, affects metabolic processes and gives rise to skeleton weakness. Bodily losses, which are obligatory, occur through the gastrointestinal tract, kidneys and the skin. A meaningful intake of calcium and vitamin D is essential for an average human. Many nutritional supplements are easily available in markets that carry vital constituents like vitamin D; which plays a role in many areas of health, including the normal absorption and utilization of calcium found in the diet as well as contributing to the normal function of our immune system. Calcium requirement increases with age, pregnancy, lactation and menopause. Loss of calcium increases rapidly in women who are post-menopausal and in men who are 55 years and beyond. Proper supplementation is required to maintain a balanced environment within the body.

Osteoporosis affects more than half of the post-menopausal women leading to bone deformities. As there is a decline in the hormone production, the bone metabolism gets affected. Therefore, the bone density is decreased leading to weaker bones that are unable to support the body's posture. A number of cases have been reported in view of calcium deficiency and fractures; especially the fracture of hip bones. Whether there is insufficiency of vitamin D due to inadequate exposure to sunlight or failure to meet the dietary requirements of calcium, both give rise to calcium deficiency.

Calcium & Vitamin D continuous consumption can help you maintain your bone mass preventing you from getting fragile, thin and weak bones and hence prevents bone deformities. Alcohol and smoking are the leading factors that are responsible for decreasing the bone mass and density.

Low bone mass can be a contributing factor to the development of fragile bones. Moreover, age, race, gender, hereditary, diet, exercise level and lifestyle habits are also responsible for changes in bone mass. Calcium & Vitamin D replaces the bone mass loss, thereby lowering the chances of osteoporosis.

4) Smooth Blood Circulation & Gout Prevention

There are two kinds of calcium; 98% of calcium is bound to the bones while the rest of the calcium is required to support heart function, circulation, nerve function and maintaining muscle tone. Lower levels of calcium cause dysfunction of such organs, predisposing to various illnesses and diseases. Calcium supplements can maintain the right amount of calcium without causing an imbalance of metabolic processes of your body. Such improvement in internal systems can reduce and prevent chances of gout.

Boron is a good choice for post-menopausal women and older men. Boron may have an impact as a hormonal stimulator that helps to increase estrogen levels which in turn maintains bone health. Estrogen related osteoporosis and testosterone losses are responsible for bone mineral density loss in females and males respectively.

5) Vitamin C, Rose hips and Acerola for Gout patients

Supplements with multiple ingredients are an excellent source of Vitamin C for your body. These supplements can provide the right amount of Rose hips and Acerola together to form the perfect combination in relieving your pain symptoms and stopping the infective causes associated with gout and other infections; providing the care you need. Mostly, lemon and other citrus flavors are added to make it easier to be taken, not causing any sort of stomach problems like indigestion or irritability.

Acerola is an organic extract. It not only has anti-oxidant properties but it acts as an antimicrobial agent.

Anti-microbial are responsible for stopping various infections encountered in everyday life. Bacterial agents are the most common ones that are found in the human body which cause diseases of various systems. Acerola has been scientifically found to be effective against the skin bacteria as well as other bacteria which cause genitourinary and lung infections.

6) Foods That Can Cause Inflammation

There are certain foods that must be avoided in order to nullify inflammation. Foods that you must not include are:
- Caffeinated teas, soda, sugar, citrus fruits, pork, processed foods, potatoes, tomatoes, all dairy products, commercial (nonorganic) eggs, all wheat products, peanut butter, shellfish, peanuts and fried foods.

7) Antioxidants, Fruits and Vegetables

The importance of eating fruits and vegetables and foods that are rich in antioxidants is obvious. Several studies over the last decade have proven the efficacy of antioxidants and green vegetables. Vegetables and fruits provide all the nutritional support that is required for the human body to operate properly. Micronutrients in fruits and vegetables strengthen our immune system to provide resistance against disabling diseases and inflammation in joints and bones that patients with gout and other types of arthritis can experience.

Antioxidants eliminate free radicals and toxins from our body. This process of cleaning harmful toxins is known as cleansing or detoxification. Antioxidants clear our body to maximize its performance.

Chapter 13: Ideal Meal Recipes for Gout Patients

Just because you have gout there is no reason for you to feel as if you have been denied everything delicious in the world. Gout is something that can and will limit your eating, but as you learn more about what food to avoid in gout diets and what can cause gout, you will realize that it is not as limited as you thought. As you put together the gout remedy report that works for you, you'll find that your gout diet treatment can actually look pretty tasty!

1) Brown Rice Sushi and Dipping Sauce

If you are someone who loves sushi, it will not escape you that some of the most famous fish for sushi, tuna and salmon, are considered high in purines and thus inappropriate for a gout-based diet. However, the truth remains that technically, sushi just refers to vinegar in rice, and there is no reason to skip the vinegary rice unless you want to!

Remember that brown rice is simply rice that still has the husks on it, and that for sushi, you should always choose brown short-grained rice. If you try to cook using long grain rice, your sushi will not stick together the way that it should.

Brown rice vegetarian sushi is a great dish to make when you want something a little luxurious, and all the extra equipment it takes is a bamboo mat designed for the purpose.

Ingredients

1 ½ cup cooked brown, short-grained rice

2-4 teaspoons of seasoned rice vinegar

2 sheets of nori

½ cucumber

¼ carrot

1 small avocado

6 tablespoons soy sauce

1-tablespoon sesame oil

1-teaspoon wasabi paste

¼ cup mirin

Allow your rice to cool to room temperature before you try to work with it.

Mix your seasoned rice vinegar into your cooked rice. The amount of vinegar that you want to put into the rice will vary from person to person. Some people like their sushi to only taste slightly of vinegar, while other people want a very intense flavor. Use your own discretion when making this decision, and keep who is eating in mind.

Lay one sheet of nori down on the bamboo mat.

Wet the nori very slightly with your fingers.

Spread a layer of rice on the nori, leaving the top ¾ inch and the bottom ¾ inch empty, but filling it out to either side.

Cut your cucumber and carrot into matchsticks

Peel your avocado and cut it into narrow thin slices.

Arrange the cucumber, the carrot, and the avocado in a row along the bottom edge of the rice. Do not overload this row of ingredients. If you put too many ingredients here, you are going to find that the sushi roll does not stay together. These are simply suggestions for ingredients to put into this sushi roll. Be creative and turn your sushi roll into real fusion cuisine. Leftover chicken fajita, pieces of pickled Japanese cabbage, and low fat cream cheese are all great choices for this recipe.

Roll the sushi from the bottom to the top, using your fingers to keep the roll tight.

Wet your fingers to seal the final free edge of nori to the rest of the roll. At this point, you should have a roll of sushi that looks like a log.

Pat the roll lightly with your fingers to make sure that it does not feel like it wants to come loose.

Repeat the process to create a second roll from your ingredients.

Use a very sharp knife to slice the sushi roll into coins that are about 1 inch thick. At this point, it is ready to eat as is, or you can continue on to make the dipping sauce as well.

Mix the soy sauce, sesame oil, wasabi paste and mirin together in a bowl. If you wish to do so, garnish it with very thinly sliced green onions. This is a great dip for sushi as well as other great Asian finger foods.

2) Applesauce Muffins

In many ways, a gout-friendly diet is one that is largely fat free. As with any change in diet, you will quickly start to miss the treats that you once had, but there are many other diet food options out there for you to try. When you are looking over diet meal plans and foods to avoid with gout, you may find that you are hungry for dessert. The best thing about applesauce muffins is that not only are they low in fat, they are intensely spicy, so you are not missing out on the flavor. As you look over gout foods to avoid, applesauce muffins will likely end up being one of your favorites dessert items!

Ingredients

1-cup flour

1½ to ¾ cup sugar, depending on how sweet you like your muffins

1-teaspoon cinnamon

½ teaspoon nutmeg

¼ teaspoon cloves

1-teaspoon baking powder

½ cup raisins

½ cup unsweetened applesauce

1/3 cup water

2/3 cup fat-free yogurt

2 eggs or 2 egg whites if you want to be very fat free

½ tsp vanilla extract

Preheat oven for 350 degrees Fahrenheit.

Mix the flour, sugar, cinnamon, nutmeg, cloves, baking powder, and raisins together in a large bowl.

Mix the applesauce, water, yogurt, eggs and vanilla extract together in another bowl, whipping until smooth.

Pour the wet ingredients into the dry ingredients.

Mix as little as possible while still mixing everything together thoroughly. The less you mix, the less you are working the gluten. If you overwork the batter, you will end up with muffins that still taste fine, but which will be more chewy and tough.

Pour the batter into a greased muffin tin. If you want to make sure that the recipe stays low in fat, use silicone muffin cups or cupcake wrappers to keep the calorie count down. If you want to add a slightly fancy touch to the muffins, make sure that you consider sprinkling some coarse sugar on top of the muffins right before they go into the oven.

Bake in the oven for about 18 minutes or until a toothpick inserted into the top of the cupcake comes out clean.

Serve warm or at room temperature.

3) Roast Root Vegetables

When you are looking to make a vegetarian main dish that is amazingly rich and flavorsome, consider roasting some root vegetables. Although this recipe is written for yams, beets and carrots, it can be adjusted to virtually any root vegetable at all.

Ingredients

2 yams

3 medium-sized beets

2-3 carrots

1 small yellow onion

2 tablespoons of olive oil

½ tablespoon garlic powder

¼ teaspoon salt

Light sour cream (optional)

Preheat your oven to 350 degrees Fahrenheit.

Peel your yams, beets, carrots and onion, and cut them into large chunks.

Throw the root vegetables into a pan.

Drizzle 2 tablespoons of olive oil over the vegetables.

Add salt and garlic powder to the vegetables.

Toss the root vegetables until everything is thoroughly coated.

Place the pan into the oven for 30 to 40 minutes or until the vegetables are cooked.

Plate immediately and serve with a dollop of light sour cream if you wish.

4) Vegetarian Lesco

As you look into gout causing foods, stop paying attention to what you cannot have and instead focus on what you can eat! Lesco is a Hungarian pepper stew, and in it's country of origin, it is served with sausage. The gout-friendly version of this dish is vegetarian, and it is quite delicious as a side dish or as a sandwich filling. Its fat comes from olive oil, which is thought by some to have some gout attack prevention qualities.

Ingredients:

2 tablespoons olive oil

1 small onion

3 yellow, orange or red peppers

1 banana pepper

2 cloves of garlic

1 tomato

Place 2 tablespoons of olive oil into a large pot and set it on the stove, heating it on medium.

Cut a small onion into thin strips, and drop them into the pot, stirring to coat the onion with the olive oil.

Cut 3 yellow, orange, or red peppers into strips and throw them into the pot as well. Do not use green peppers for this purpose, as they are too bitter.

Cut 1 banana pepper into thin rings, and throw it into the pot.

Mince 2 cloves of garlic and add it to the pot.

Dice 1 tomato, and add it to the pot.

Pour 1 8-oz can of tomato sauce into the pot.

Pour cups of water into the pot until all of the ingredients are covered.

Stir the ingredients together, and then turn the burner up to high.

Let the ingredients cook together for at least 1 hour, returning to stir occasionally and to add more water to the pot as necessary. Do not let the lesco boil dry.

Allow the lesco to cook until it is of a stew-like consistency, and then serve.

5) Turkey Burgers

If you are not actually a vegetarian, there is likely a chance that you have enjoyed a burger or two...or three or four! Burgers are great, but if you get them from the restaurant, they are full of red meat, which is a real problem if you are on a low-purine diet. This is where turkey burgers come to the rescue. A turkey burger is not made of red meat, but it can be delicious in its own right. Take a moment to consider how to make a truly delicious turkey burger.

Ingredients

1-pound ground turkey

Sprinkle of whole-wheat breadcrumbs or wet textured vegetable protein

¼ minced white onion

1 egg white

1 minced garlic clove

Salt and black pepper

Whole-wheat hamburger buns

Combine all of the ingredients together in a large bowl and mix them thoroughly. The amount of salt and pepper you add is up to you, but if you are feeling conservative, a light sprinkle of each will do.

Shape the mixture into patties with your hands. You can get 2 large patties or 4 small patties from this recipe.

Grill the turkey patties over a medium-high heat in a non-stick skillet until the turkey is cooked all the way through. You cannot

139

serve turkey rare the way that you can with beef, so be certain that the patties are well done,

Place the patties on whole-wheat hamburger buns and add condiments as you please.

6) Lentil or Rice Burgers

When you want to enjoy something that is both healthy and flavorsome, consider lentil burgers. Lentil burgers give you plenty of nutrients without the fat and calorific load of meat burgers of any variety. This lentil burger is a fantastic choice when you are looking to cut calories and to make sure that you are still satisfied at the end of the meal. While you can of course top it with regular hamburger toppings, this burger goes quite well with salsa and a small amount of low-fat cheese.

While lentils are high in purines, some people report being able to eat them with no issues. If you are leery about lentils, consider replacing them with cooked rice in the recipe.

Ingredients

1-2 slices of whole-wheat bread

3 cups cooked red lentils or rice

3 eggs

½ teaspoon of salt

1-teaspoon garlic powder

1-tablespoon olive oil

Toast 1-2 slices of whole-wheat bread. When the bread pops, tear it into smallish breadcrumbs, and set it aside.

Mix your cooked red lentils, eggs, garlic powder, and salt very thoroughly, smashing them together until they are quite runny. If you have a food processor, this can make the process much easier. Do not worry if you still see whole lentils in the mixture as long as the texture is even.

Stir in the breadcrumbs.

Cover the bowl and leave it alone for ten minutes. This allows the mixture to come together a little more. You can add more breadcrumbs for a more sturdy texture if you prefer.

Split the mixture into 4 to 6 patties.

Pour 1 tablespoon of olive oil into a skillet and heat it over medium-low heat.

Lay the patties into the skillet and cover them with a lid, allowing them to cook for about 8 minutes.

Flip the patties and cook for another 5 to 7 minutes.

At this point, the patties are ready to be placed on whole wheat hamburger buns and served.

7) Sweet Potato Fries

When you are on a gout-friendly diet, you will discover that one thing that you might miss are potatoes. Potatoes are often considered an undesirable food for gout diets because they are full of empty calories, starch and sugar. However, the potato's relative, the sweet potato, is actually not only fine, but quite desirable! Sweet potatoes are full of vitamin A, they are full of anti-oxidants, and they provide a colorful splash to your diet. When you are looking for something to dip into ketchup and to accompany your gout-friendly burgers, consider what sweet potato fries can do for you.

Ingredients

3 large sweet potatoes

2 tablespoons olive oil

1 ½ teaspoon salt

½ teaspoon parsley

1 tablespoon of your favorite spice or spice mix, Cajun seasoning, mace, Bay seasoning, chipotle seasoning or allspice work well (Optional)

Preheat your oven to 400 degrees Fahrenheit

Peel your potatoes and cut them into wedges. If the wedges are very long, cut them in half.

Throw all of your ingredients into a large bowl and stir to cover the wedges in the oil and spice mixture.

Lay the wedges on a non-stick baking sheet or a baking sheet covered with aluminum foil in a single layer.

Place the baking sheet into the oven and bake for 30 minutes, removing the fries to turn them at the 15-minute mark.

Remove the fries from the oven and enjoy with ketchup, mustard, horseradish or your favorite condiment.

8) Black Cherry Juice

While you are cutting back on alcohol and probably on sodas as well, you may be really craving something sweet to drink. The answer can be found in black cherry juice. Black cherries have been shown to remove uric acid from the system, and if you make your own, you can ensure that there are no fillers or other harmful chemicals in them. Black cherry juice is on the expensive side to make yourself, but once you try it, you are not going to be satisfied with what you get at the store anymore! While you can use frozen black cherries for this purpose, fresh black cherries are much more delicious.

Cherry juice for gout is often included on a long list of gout medications, so when you are dealing with symptoms of gout in foot areas, you will find that this might be the perfect drink for you to make and then to freeze for later consumption. If you have never tried fresh, home-made cherry juice, now is the time to start. If you do not have the time or the inclination to make your own cherry juice, it is a good idea to consider black cherry supplements, which are available from most alternative health and vitamin stores.

Ingredients

2-3 cups pitted black cherries

2 cups of water

2 tablespoons Splenda or other low-fat sweetener (optional)

Combine all of the ingredients in a pan and bring to the boil, stirring occasionally.

When the cherries reach the boiling point, turn down the heat and simmer for another 10 minutes. Do not cover the cherries.

Mash the cherries until they are completely pulped. You can do this with a pestle, a large spatula or a potato masher.

Place a fine sieve over a bowl.

Pour the cherry mixture into the sieve.

Use a spoon to smash the cherries down until all of the liquid is drained into the bowl below.

Allow the cherry juice to cool completely in the refrigerator. You can keep the cherry juice for two to three days, or you can freeze it to save it for later.

Drink as is, or thin the solution with water.

9) Chicken Fajita

As you get away from a high purine diet and learn more about the causes of gout, you will find that you are eating a lot of chicken! The truth of the matter is that is that chicken does not have to be as dull as you were afraid of.

Chicken that is marinated, as in the case of these chicken fajitas, are quite tasty, and you'll find that as you realize what causes gout that it is possible to eat quite well. As you learn more about what the cause for gout is, you will discover more and more of these great recipes.

Ingredients

1½ to 2 pounds chicken breast

4 tablespoons olive oil, divided

2 tablespoons lime juice

1-teaspoon honey

½ teaspoon salt

½ teaspoon cumin

½ teaspoon chili

½ teaspoon paprika

1-4 cloves minced garlic

1 small onion

2 green peppers

Slice all of the chicken breast into strips and throw them into a re-sealable bag or a bowl with a lid.

Add the limejuice, 3 tablespoons of olive oil, the honey, all of the spices and the garlic to the chicken.

Seal the container and let it sit anywhere from 1 hour to overnight in the refrigerator. The longer you let it sit, the more flavorsome this recipe is.

Pour the marinated chicken into a skillet and cook on medium high until meat is lightly browned and cooked all the way through.

Remove the chicken from the pan and place it on a paper towel to drain.

Slice 1 small onion into strips as you get ready to start the meal.

Heat 1 teaspoon of olive oil in the same skillet. If you are very worried about fat consumption, skip the olive oil and simply cook the onion in the oil from the marinated chicken.

Brown the onion in the skillet, stirring regularly until the onion strips are soft.

Slice 2 green peppers into strips when you are ready to start cooking the meal.

Turn to low or medium low, and cook the green peppers and onions until they are soft.

Stir in the chicken, and mix until everything is equally warm.

Remove from heat and serve on brown rice, on whole-wheat tortillas or on whole-wheat bread.

10) Vegetarian Vegetable Soup

One of the unexpected things that might surprise you when you are looking at foods to avoid when you have gout is that you have to be careful with soup. Even soup that is low in fat is frequently made with chicken stock, and chicken stock is often cooked from bones and connective tissue, which are full of purines and high on the list of foods to avoid if you have gout. When it comes to gout, uric acid and the foods to avoid for arthritis in general are very high on the list of things for you to be thinking about. Check out foods to avoid gout, and learn more about how to cook well with this fantastic basic vegetable soup recipe.

This soup is a fantastic choice when you are looking at throwing something together for a cold day, and you'll find that as with a number of different soups, it gets better and better as you heat it up. To turn this simple soup into a light meal, consider adding a whole-wheat roll spread with some reduced fat butter.

Ingredients

1-tablespoon olive oil

1 small white onion

2 carrots

1 small zucchini

1 stalk of celery

1 large tomato

1-teaspoon salt

1-teaspoon oregano

1-teaspoon black pepper

3 16- ounce cans of vegetable broth

1 8-ounce can of tomato paste

Heat 1 tablespoon of olive oil in a large pot.

Slice 1 small white onion into strips, and brown gently over a medium heat.

Slice two peeled carrots into thin coins, and throw them into the pot.

Slice 1 small zucchini into thin coins, and throw them into the pot. For some visual variety, peel the zucchini in alternating stripes, letting the white of the zucchini's flesh contrast with the dark of the peel. This makes for a lovely contrast in the soup.

Cut 2 celery stalks into small pieces and throw the pieces in.

Dice 1 large tomato, and throw the pieces into the pot.

Add all of the spices, the broth and the tomato paste.

Add enough water to cover everything.

Bring to a light boil, and then turn down to a low simmer.

Cook until the ingredients are soft. This usually takes between 30 minutes to an hour, but you can cook to your taste. Some people really love a very mushy soup, while others like a little bit of toughness to their vegetables.

Serve hot with a slice of whole-wheat toast. Some people also throw a handful of whole-wheat pasta into the soup as it is cooking.

11) Simple Risotto

As you are struggling with the causes of gout and what not to eat if you have gout, you will find yourself craving simple, homey dishes that you can prepare with the ingredients you have to hand. When you are wondering what gout diet to do, take a moment to learn to cook risotto.

This classic French dish is often a little intimidating, but the truth is that it is quite easy, and thanks to the starch in short-grain rice, it is also quite rich without having the fat that often goes with a really tasty dish. Risotto takes time, but the end results are worth it. While you are struggling with your gout medication, learn to make risotto that will serve as an excellent comfort food and a great food for your entire family in general.

Ingredients

1-tablespoon olive oil

1 small white onion

1 cup of any short grain rice, though Arborio rice is the best for this purpose

4 cups of vegetable broth

Salt and pepper

Heat 1 tablespoon of olive oil in a large skillet.

Slice the small white onion into strips.

Sauté the onion in the skillet until it is brown and soft.

Turn the heat to medium-low

Add the raw rice to the skillet, stirring with a wooden spoon until every grain is covered with oil.

Heat the vegetable broth in another pot, and allow it to rise to a steady low simmer.

Add a ladle of the vegetable broth to the heating rice, stirring thoroughly so that the broth is completely absorbed.

Stir until you can no longer see any broth in the rice.

Add ladles of broth and stir them in until all of the broth has been absorbed. At this point, the rice will have released its starch, creating a texture that is very rich and creamy despite not having a bit of animal fat or dairy in it.

Serve hot, adding salt and pepper to suit individual tastes. Some people add a sprinkle of parsley over the top to add some color, while other people add a bit of low-fat Parmesan cheese.

12) Skordalia

When you are looking at what gout is and what causes it, and when you are busy concerning yourself with foods to avoid in gout and gout treatment foods, you might start craving something that feels a bit like junk food. With gout symptoms and causes and home remedies, gout is something that can seriously make you long for some easy chips and dip.

While a lot of dips are high on the list of gout foods to avoid, you will find that this Greek dip is perfect as a low-fat, low purine snack. Remember that potatoes can be a risky food for some people, but if you eat a smaller amount, you should be fine. Skordalia is a traditional Greek dish, and it can be used as a sandwich spread or a dip. It is strongly flavored and a perfect choice when you are looking for the perfect snack.

Ingredients

2 russet potatoes

8 cloves of garlic

½ cup olive oil

1-teaspoon salt

1-2 tablespoons of lemon juice

Peel and boil the russet potatoes until they are soft, and then set them aside.

Peel and mince the garlic. If you want a milder taste, simply crush the garlic very thoroughly.

Place the potatoes and garlic in a large bowl.

Add olive oil, salt and lemon juice.

Mash thoroughly with a potato masher until the skordalia is smooth. If you want the texture to be a little silkier, add some water.

Serve cool, with pita chips or with sliced vegetables.

13) Orange Sesame Chicken

Just because you are on a gout-friendly diet does not mean that you need to be in a situation where all of your foods are dull. Learning to cook with a worldwide flavor will quickly catch your interest, and as you learn what foods have uric acid and which gout treatment diet works well for you, you will quickly realize that it does not all have to be bland!

This orange-sesame dish comes from general Chinese-American cuisine, and it contains none of the foods that you have to avoid for gout. As you look into a low purine diet for gout and start looking at food to avoid, this is one recipe that is sure to get revisited time and time again.

<u>Ingredients</u>

2 tablespoons sesame oil, divided

1½-2 pounds chicken breast

3 cloves garlic

1 inch of fresh ginger

2 carrots

1-2 cups peas

¼ cup apple cider vinegar

¾ cup orange juice

2-3 tablespoons soy sauce

1-tablespoon sugar

1-tablespoon honey

1-tablespoons cornstarch

Heat 1 tablespoon of sesame oil on the frying pan on medium-high heat. Remember that a great trick for getting the most flavor out of your oil in stir-fry situations is to start with a cold pan, to warm it, and then to add room-temperature oil to it. Be careful of splatters if you do this!

Slice the chicken breast into strips.

Mince your garlic thoroughly.

Peel and mince your ginger thoroughly. If you are not sure that you want all that much ginger flavor in your chicken, you can simply cut the ginger into coins, and fish it out after the cooking is done.

Add the chicken breast, garlic and ginger to the pan, cooking until the chicken is thoroughly cooked and beginning to brown. Set the chicken aside on a plate.

Peel and slice your carrots into thin coins.

Pour 1 tablespoon of sesame oil into the pan and cook your carrots on a medium heat until they soften up.

Add the chicken back to the skillet.

Add peas to the skillet.

Pour orange juice, vinegar, soy sauce and cornstarch into a bowl and mix them until they are smooth.

Pour the sweet orange juice mixture over the contents of the skillet.

Cook for another 3 to 5 minutes over a medium heat. Stir with a paddle or wooden spoon to make sure that everything is coated thoroughly with the mixture.

Serve over brown rice or eat on its own. You can also sprinkle the top of the dish with toasted sesame seeds for visual variety.

14) Honey Balsamic Vinaigrette

As you start eating the gout diet, getting involved with gout treatment medications and learning about gout home remedies, you are going to get pretty tired of salads. People will start telling you that you can always have salad, but let's face it, if you were really in the mood for a juicy steak or a tuna sandwich, salad is a pretty poor substitute.

However, remember that salad on its own can be pretty awesome if you learn to make your own gout-safe dressings. When it comes to gout, what foods to avoid are important, but you also need to think about making the foods that you can eat even better. This honey balsamic vinaigrette is the perfect way to spice up a boring salad, and it definitely beats reaching for that bottle of ranch or French dressing one more time!

Ingredients

3 tablespoons balsamic vinegar

1 ½ tablespoons honey

¼ cup cold-pressed olive oil

¼ teaspoon coarse sea salt

¼ teaspoon crushed black pepper

Throw all of the ingredients together into a bowl.

Whisk thoroughly and serve on your favorite salads. This salad dressing is a great choice when you want to add a richer flavor to salads that are otherwise a little bit dull. For a little more zing, add more crushed black pepper to the mix.

Use sparingly as you add this to your salad. A little bit of this dressing goes a long way. If it is a little intense, you can thin it with water, though if you want something that is a little more intense, think about adding more honey or even some red pepper flakes.

15) Chai Tea

As you remove purine rich foods from your diet, and as you move forward towards finding the best home remedies for arthritis, you may find that you are in a spot where you miss sweet drinks. Some people are triggered by carbonated beverages, and when you are looking for something more interesting than water, you should think about chai tea.

Chai tea is an Indian recipe that uses spices and milk in black tea to create a warm and deliciously sweet drink. The ginger in the tea makes for an excellent gout remedy, and though it is not considered a standard uric acid treatment, it's a great beverage all on its own. Don't let yourself get so overwhelmed with low purine foods and learning about gout symptoms food that you end up denying yourself anything flavorsome!

<u>Ingredients</u>

2 cups of water

¼ cup honey

5 bags of black tea

1 cinnamon stick

4 whole cloves

¼ teaspoon of ginger

1/3 teaspoons ground cardamom

2 cups rice milk or almond milk

Boil 2 cups of water in a small pot.

Stir in all of the spices and the honey.

Remove the tags from the black tea bag, and toss them in as well.

Simmer everything for 5 minutes. You can simmer for 6 to 7 if you wish, but this makes for a very powerful black tea taste.

Remove the teabags from the liquid.

Add the rice milk or the almond milk. Both of these milks are great substitutes if you find that your gout attacks are sensitive to dairy.

Raise the temperature to high, and bring to the boil. Watch the pot, because boiling happens rather quickly.

Remove the pot from the stove.

Remove the cinnamon stick, and reuse it later if you wish to do so.

Serve as is, or, for a more professional presentation, simply strain it through a filter, a strainer or even cheesecloth.

16) Garlic Roasted in Balsamic Vinegar

When you are looking for a way to add savor to your meals but you don't want to pile on the fat or to mess with fat substitutes, you will find that vinegar and garlic are your friends. These are two flavors that are so closely related to meat and when they are combined you will find that they make an excellent garnish.

This recipe relies on garlic and balsamic vinegar coming together into a rich topping that goes well on pasta, on whole-wheat bread and on fish. It is an excellent choice when you feel as if you have been missing out on rich flavors.

Ingredients

4 heads of garlic

½ cup balsamic vinegar

½ cup olive oil

Separate and peel every single clove of garlic from the four heads, and cut off the tough ends. To make this process simpler, separate the individual cloves and place them between two bowls, closing them inside. Shake the two bowls vigorously, and most of the papery peel will just fall off.

Place the garlic cloves in a small saucepan, and cover them with the balsamic vinegar and the olive oil.

Turn the stove to medium-low.

Stir the garlic constantly for forty minutes or until the garlic yields to light pressure.

Remove the garlic from the stove and drain away the liquid. If you are feeling thrifty, you can use the liquid to fry something else or even to make a truly powerful pasta sauce.

Serve the balsamic vinegar infused garlic slightly warm or at room temperature. One great way to serve this item is to simply spread it on a slice of whole-wheat bread and then to sprinkle it with a low fat cheese.

17) Chicken Salad

When you are in a spot where you want to create a large batch of something for a picnic, or you just want something you can eat for a little while, chicken salad is a great choice. It makes an excellent side dish or sandwich filling, and once you make it, you can adjust the recipe as you see fit to make sure that you have something that you will always find tasty. This recipe is easily doubled or tripled or halved to create something that suits your needs for the day.

Ingredients

½ pound cooked chicken breast

½ cup grapes

¼ small red onion

1 stalk celery

2 tablespoons dried parsley

4 tablespoons low fat mayonnaise

3 tablespoons fat free Greek yogurt

1-tablespoon mustard

1-tablespoon apple cider vinegar

Salt and pepper

Shred the chicken breast finely using your fingers or a fork.

Dice the grapes, onion and celery.

Mix the chicken breast, grapes, onion and celery into a bowl.

Add the parsley, mayonnaise, yogurt, mustard, and apple cider vinegar.

Mix all of the ingredients thoroughly, until everything is covered.

Set aside in the refrigerator for at least an hour. If you leave it overnight, the flavors will blend more completely.

Add salt and pepper to taste. This recipe does particularly well on a whole-wheat roll.

18) Tomato Salsa

When you are eating a low fat and low purine diet, it is easy to forget that strong flavors are an option. However, if you are looking for something tangy and spicy, you'll find that a great tomato salsa can really liven things up. Use this tomato salsa as a topping for your favorite starches, to eat with pita chips or even as a delicious sandwich topping.

You may think that salsa is dull, but the truth is that until you have had it homemade, you don't know what you are missing!

<u>Ingredients</u>

3 tomatoes

1 small red onion

1 jalapeno

4-5 tablespoons lime juice

½ cup chopped cilantro

Dice your tomatoes roughly and place them in a glass bowl. A glass bowl is the best choice when you are preparing something as acidic as tomatoes, as it will not change the taste.

Mince your small red onion, and add it to the tomato.

Slit the jalapeno in half, remove the stem and rinse out the seeds.

Mince the jalapeno, and add it to the salsa. If you want a spicier salsa, add a Serrano pepper or a chili pepper to the mix.

Add ½ cup of chopped cilantro.

Mix thoroughly.

Cover the bowl, and refrigerate for at least an hour. The longer you let the bowl of salsa sit, the more the flavors will blend and the better it will become.

19) Pita Chips

After hearing all about the different things that you can use as dips and condiments, you may be feeling a little nervous about what you can use them with! Pita chips are a great choice when you are looking at finding something that is healthy and delicious. They are quick, and they can easily be added to any menu where you want something light and snack-like.

When you are thinking about making something special for a party, you can double this recipe easily. Basically, you simply need one tablespoon of oil for each pita that you decide to use. To cut back on the oil that is used, use a silicone brush to sweep it onto the pitas.

Ingredients

3 pitas

3 tablespoons of olive oil

Garlic powder

Preheat the oven to 375 degrees Fahrenheit.

Rub olive oil onto both sides of each pita.

Lay the pitas on baking sheets.

Use a pizza cutter to cut each pita into 8 triangular wedges.

Sprinkle the pita wedges with garlic powder. Add salt and pepper if desired.

Bake in the oven for 10 minutes or until crisp.

Remove from the oven and allow to cool slightly before consuming.

20) Grilled Chicken Sandwich

When you are looking at low fat recipes, you may be fairly startled to see how often chicken breast comes up. The truth is that chicken breast is a low fat protein that is relatively inoffensive as far as taste goes. That is why if you prepare chicken breast the way that you prepare your steak, you are going to be disappointed. Chicken breast, especially chicken breast that is purchased from a grocery store rather than a farmer or a farmer's market, is relatively tasteless.

Marinating your chicken breast gives it a fantastic flavor and it can make an excellent basis for a chicken sandwich with all of the trimmings. This is a deluxe chicken sandwich that is sure to make you savor every bite!

Ingredients

2 raw chicken breasts

2 tablespoons honey

1-tablespoon olive oil

2 tablespoons balsamic vinegar

2 cloves garlic

¼ teaspoon salt

Whole-wheat buns

Lettuce leaves

Tomato slices

Onion slices

Condiments

Throw the chicken breasts into a re-sealable plastic bag with the honey, the olive oil, and the balsamic vinegar.

Peel your garlic cloves and mince them up.

Add the garlic cloves to the bag.

Put the bag containing the chicken and the spices into the refrigerator and leave them overnight for the best taste. You can take them out in an hour or two, but the flavor will not be as bold.

Heat a pan on the stove until it is warm to the touch.

Remove the chicken breasts from the bag, and lay them on the pan.

Cook the chicken on high heat until both sides are seared.

Turn the heat down to medium low and cover until the chicken is thoroughly cooked. This may take between 5 and 10 minutes depending on your stove.

Toast your whole-wheat buns if desired.

Lay the chicken breasts on the buns.

Top with lettuce, tomato and onion slices, and add condiments as you wish. If you are trying to keep things low fat, use low-fat mayo and low-fat ketchup.

Chapter 14: Alternative Medicine

We have learned plenty about gout and its treatment. Now, let's talk about some alternative remedies which can be used along with the ongoing treatment. It's recommended to use them in combination and don't replace the conventional therapy. The most commonly used remedies are as follows:

Vitamin C
Vitamin C is not only a strong antioxidant but also beneficial to lower uric acid levels in the body. Vitamin C is effective in low doses and must be avoided in high doses, which can cause an increase in uric acid levels in the body. Patients with kidney problems are not recommended to take vitamin C. Dosages above 2,000mg per day can cause gastric disturbances and high uric acid levels. 500mg once daily is recommended to lower uric acid levels. Consult with your doctor before taking any vitamin C.

Cherries
Cherries are beneficial in lowering uric acid levels in the body. One cup is recommended to fill the need. They can also be diluted with water to make juice. Besides cherries, dark colored fruits like blue berries and raspberries are also effective in the treatment of gout. Cherries being anti-inflammatory reduce inflammation in the body.

Coffee
Caffeinated and non-caffeinated coffee have shown remarkable results in lowering uric acid levels. Although, there is not much scientific explanation available for this phenomena but it sounds quite promising in future treatment.

Vitamin E
Vitamin E is not only an antioxidant but also an anti-inflammatory in nature .Therefore, 400IU daily might help to improve the situation and can prevent extreme pain flares when an attack occurs.

Bromelain
It's a bioflavanoid only found in pineapple. It's suggested to take 400-500mg during a gout attack. Being an anti-inflammatory agent, it reduces inflammation in the body. It's advised to take bromelin on an empty stomach otherwise it will work as a digestive enzyme.

Quercetin
Unlike bromelin, Quercetin is a bioflavonoids which is abundantly present in apples, berries, green and black tea, broccoli, cauliflower, cabbage, onion and leafy vegetables. It is not only an anti-inflammatory, but also reduces the formation of uric acid in the body. It also helps in excretion of uric acid. It is compared with Allopurinol in efficacy to inhibit production of uric acid. Its recommended dose is 200-4000mg between meals.

Flax Seed Oil
Flax seed oil is also called linseed oil and is very beneficial for gout patients. They contain more omega-3 and available in the form of soft gel omega-3 and omega--6 capsules. They are anti-inflammatory in nature and reduce inflammation in the body. The recommended daily dose is 1cap daily with a lot of water. It can also be sprinkled on yogurt or salad directly. It's rich in alpha-linolenic acid, which is beneficial in heart disease.

These supplements should only be taken after consultation with your doctor. Many of these have shown beneficial results in improving overall wellbeing along with conventional therapy used to treat gout.

Chapter 15: Additional Medication Information

1) General information on NSAIDs

Under certain circumstances medication for Gout, especially NSAIDs, (non-steroidal anti-inflammatory drugs) can lead to fatal disorders like bleeding and ulcers. Such disorders can take place during anytime of medication use without any prior signs or symptoms.

Nevertheless, such dangerous side-effects of NSAIDs mostly happen as a result of some specific activities/situations that include:
- Longer or over consumption of medication,
- Alcoholism or substance (drug) abuse,
- Older age (intake of any medication should be kept under critical check in old age patients),
- Smoking (smoking is injurious to health in multiple ways & can lead to life threatening illnesses),
- Intake of medication that belongs to drug classes named "anticoagulants" and "corticosteroids".
NSAIDs based medications should be taken at lowest dose possible for gout treatment follow exact prescription of your physician and last but not least, use NSAIDs for shortest time needed.

There are also some other medical conditions that demand serious precautions while taking NSAIDs like; allergic reactions to aspirin, hives, heart by-pass burger, pregnancy and lactation (particularly at third trimester in pregnancy) and asthma attack.

Physicians should be well aware of your medical history and medications that you have been using, to safely prescribe you any NSAIDs drugs. Some patients do not bother informing their physician about over-the-counter drugs or vitamin/herb supplementation use. It can be harmful as NSAIDs can interact with some other medications that may lead to serious side-effects.

Some Serious/harmful side-effects related to NSAIDs are:

-High blood pressure, Stroke, heart attack
- Anemia (low red blood cell count)
- Gastrointestinal disorders like ulcers and bleeding (in the stomach and intestine)
- Heart failure that can occur as a result of fluid retention (body swelling)
- Severe skin and life threatening allergic reactions
- Liver failure and other liver-related complications
- Kidney failure and other kidney-related complications
- Increase in asthma attacks in patients already suffering with asthma.

Some common but less harmful side-effects related to NSAIDs are:

-Heartburn, nausea, vomiting, gas, diarrhea, stomach pain, dizziness, and constipation.

Certain Conditions That You Must Consider As Emergencies

There are certain conditions and symptoms that require immediate attention and a halt in medication until professionally advised. Conditions that demand serious attention includes; weakness and pain in certain parts of the body (arms, hands, legs, feet), swelling on face, swelling on throat, shortness of breath or any breathing difficulties, chest pain, nausea, yellowish eyes, unusual weight increase or weight loss, vomiting with blood in it, itching or rash on skin, and abdominal pain. You must respond quickly and need to contact your health care provider for instructions.

The above mentioned medical conditions are not complete by any means and more side-effects can be experienced with the frequent use of NSAIDs drugs. Not all drugs in this class can cause each of the above mentioned disorders. For example, aspirin does belong to NSAIDs group, but it will not put you in danger to have cardiac arrest, heart attack or stroke. Nonetheless, aspirin can certainly cause bleeding and ulcer in intestine and stomach. Many practitioners allow intake of NSAIDs in low doses up to 10 days or less even without prescription (over-the-counter). A brief from a healthcare professional or a pharmacist can be handy indeed.

2) Specific NSAIDs

Aspirin

Indomethacin

Ketoprofen

Mefenamic Acid

Meloxicam

3) Guidelines For Medication

Useful Information to Maximize the Purpose of Medications: After years of research and clinical trials in the pharmaceutical industry, scientists have proposed parameters to maximize the benefits of medications.

These guidelines are multi-purpose; to promote healthy lifestyle and demoralize careless and unhealthy habits. Following are some guidelines that everyone should follow to ensure the best outcome from treatment and medication:

- Avoid drinking alcohol. However, if you are addicted to it and cannot leave it completely then make sure you consume it in small quantity. Alcoholism and substance abuse are seriously injurious to health, especially in old age.

- Always follow your physician's instructions carefully.
- Some medications can cause gastrointestinal problems so it is better to take medicines with either milk or citrus foods to minimize the negative impact.

- Hydrate your body more than usual, like 2 to 3 liters of water everyday unless you are on a particular diet or restricted by your doctor.

- Keep in mind that some medications can cause dizziness, so be cautious to take medicines when you need to drive or have to perform any particular task that require alertness and concentration.

- Intake of food in small proportions is ideal with NSAIDs, analgesics and uric acid lowering agents. This may help reduce heartburn. Additionally, chewing gums and lozenges can also help.
- Weight gain can be easily associated with long-term use of several medicines. Ideally, weigh yourself weekly and let your doctor know about it. This way, your doctor can analyze and change prescription if required.

Ideal Readings & Suggested Studies

1. Name of the Book: Gout: *The Patrician Malady*

Written by Roy Porter, G. S. Rousseau.
Overview of the book: Gout has interested medical writers and cultural commentators from the time of Ancient Greece. Historically seen as a disease afflicting upper-class males of superior wit, genius and creativity, it has included among its sufferers Erasmus, the Medici, Edward Gibbon, Samuel Johnson, Immanuel Kant and Robert Browning. Gout has also been the subject of medical folklore, viewed as a disease that protects its sufferers and assure long life.

This book investigates the history of gout and through it, offers a perspective on medical and social history, sex, prejudice and class and explains why gout was gender specific. The authors investigate medical thinking about gout through the ages, from Hippocrates and Galen through Paracelsus and Harvey to Archibald Garrod in the Victorian era and beyond. They discuss the cultural, moral, religious and personal qualities associated with gout, examining social commentary, personal writings, cartoons and visual arts, and imaginative literature (including novels of Dickens, Thackeray and Joseph Conrad).

2. Name of the Book: *Gout*

By Llewellyn Jones Llewellyn, in August 2012.
Overview of this book: Unlike some other reproductions of classic texts. (1) We have not used OCR (Optical Character Recognition), as this leads to bad quality books with introduced typos. (2) In books where there are images such as portraits, maps, sketches etc. we have endeavored to keep the quality of these images, so they represent accurately the original artifact. Although occasionally there may be certain imperfections with

these old texts, we feel they deserve to be made available for future generations to enjoy.

3. Name of the Book: *Galileo's Gout: Science in an Age of Endarkenment,* **by Gerald Weissmann.**

Overview of this book: My hopes for this book ran high: the creation of the word "endarkenment" was promising. The introduction and first chapter were also promising, as they appeared to be discussing the issue of science in an age of irrationality and pseudoscience. It turns out, however, that the book is much more a history of urology than a discussion of the topic of irrational belief and psuedoscience. While it was possibly a decent book on the topic, urology is not an area I spend a great deal of time reading about, and I would have liked a more genuine description of what the book really was.

4. Name of the book: *Getting Rid of Gout*: **by Bryan Emmerson.**

Overview of this book: Anyone suffering from this traumatic arthritic condition will fully appreciate the new edition of Getting Rid of Gout. Included in the new sections are updated dietary guidelines, including current research on the role of diet in preventing gout, and a description of the new medications available for its treatment.
Written in an understandable and sympathetic manner with the aid of diagrams and cartoons ,Getting Rid of Gout offers sensible advice and dispels the popular fallacies about the nature and causes of gout.

5. Name of the book: *Meditations on Gout*: **With a Consideration of Its Cure Through the use of Wine: by George H. Ellwanger in the year 2003.**

Overview of this book: This scarce antiquarian book is a facsimile reprint of the original. Due to its age, it may contain imperfections such as marks, notations, marginalia and flawed pages. Because we believe this work is culturally important, we have made it available as part of our commitment for protecting, preserving, and promoting the world's literature in affordable, high quality, modern editions that are true to the original work.

References

* Gout & Its Cure:
Written by J. C. Burnett.
* The Treatment of Modern Western Medical Diseases with
Chinese Medicine: A textbook and clinical manual.
Written by Bob Flaws, and Philippe Sionneau,
* J & B Clinical Card: Gout
Written by Marc Miller.
* Prescription for Natural Cures: A Self-Care Guide for Treating
Health Problems with natural remedies.
 Written by James F. Balch, Mark Stengler.
* Gout, Its Cause, Nature, and Treatment: With Directions for the
Regulation of the Diet
Written by John Parkin, Kessinger Publishing, 01-Feb-2009.
* Concise Clinical Pharmacology:
Written by Ben Greenstein, Adam Greenstein.
* Medicine at a Glance:
 Edited by Patrick Davey.
* Kochar's Clinical Medicine for Students:
 Edited by Dario M. Torre, Geoffrey C. Lamb, Jerome Van
Ruiswyk, Ralph M. Schapira.
* Internal Medicine Essentials for Clerkship Students 2
 Edited by Patrick Craig Alguire.
* Rheumatism and Gout:
By Francis Le Roy Satterlee.
* Color Atlas of Pharmacology:
 Edited by Heinz Lüllmann.
* Bone and Joint Disorders
 By Francis A. Burgener, Martti Kormano.
* Essential Evidence: Medicine that Matters
 By David Slawson, Allen Shaughnessy, Mark Ebell, Henry
Barry.
* Diseases of the Kidney and Urinary Tract
 Edited by Robert W. Schrier.

* The Netter Collection of Medical Illustrations - Integumentary System:
 By Bryan E. Anderson.
* Food and Nutrition:
Enzymes to gout.
* Rheumatology: Diagnosis and Therapeutics
 Edited by John J. Cush, Arthur Kavanaugh, Charles Michael Stein.

Published by IMB Publishing 2014

Made in the USA
Coppell, TX
17 October 2023

22977251R00095